The Diabetic Athlete

Sheri Colberg, PhD
Old Dominion University

Human Kinetics

Library of Congress Cataloging-in-Publication Data

Colberg, Sheri R., 1963-
    The diabetic athlete / Sheri R. Colberg.
      p. cm
    Includes bibliographical references and index.
    ISBN 0-7360-3271-1
      1. Diabetic athletes. 2. Diabetes--Exercise therapy. I. Title.

    RC660 .C4746 2001
    616.4'62'0088796   00-031907

ISBN: 0-7360-3271-1

Acquisitions Editor: Martin Barnard; **Developmental Editor:** Cassandra Mitchell; **Assistant Editor:** Wendy McLaughlin; **Copyeditor:** Jan Feeney; **Proofreader:** Erin Cler; **Indexer:** Sheri Colberg; **Graphic Designer:** Stuart Cartwright; **Graphic Artist:** Tara Welsch; **Photo Manager:** Clark Brooks; **Cover Designer:** Keith Blomberg; **Photographer (cover):** Tom Roberts; Actionimages; **Photographer (interior):** Tom Roberts unless otherwise noted; **Art Manager:** Craig Newsom; **Illustrator:** Accurate Art; **Printer:** United Graphics

Note: Photos used in this book are for illustration purposes only and do not in any manner imply any medical conditions of the individuals featured.

Human Kinetics books are available at special discounts for bulk purchase. Special editions or book excerpts can also be created to specification. For details, contact the Special Sales Manager at Human Kinetics.

Printed in the United States of America   10 9 8 7 6 5 4 3

Human Kinetics
Web site: www.HumanKinetics.com

United States: Human Kinetics
P.O. Box 5076
Champaign, IL 61825-5076
800-747-4457
e-mail: humank@hkusa.com

Canada: Human Kinetics
475 Devonshire Road, Unit 100
Windsor, ON N8Y 2L5
800-465-7301 (in Canada only)
e-mail: orders@hkcanada.com

Europe: Human Kinetics
107 Bradford Road
Stanningley
Leeds LS28 6AT, United Kingdom
+44 (0)113 255 5665
e-mail: hk@hkeurope.com

Australia: Human Kinetics
57A Price Avenue
Lower Mitcham, South Australia 5062
08 8277 1555
e-mail: liahka@senet.com.au

New Zealand: Human Kinetics
P.O. Box 105-231, Auckland Central
09-523-3462
e-mail: hkp@ihug.co.nz

This book is dedicated to my family members who have loved and supported me unconditionally during its creation. My wonderful husband, Ray Ochs, has truly been a ray of sunshine and a blessing in my life. My three delightful sons, Alex, Anton, and Ray-J, have kept me focused on what is really important in life and have kept me playing. My ever-supportive mother, Karen Colberg, has shown me how to be a good parent with her actions. My father, Don Colberg, has inspired me with his love of books.

contents

foreword

Given the problems associated with the long-term complications of diabetes, along with the inherent risks in some sports, people with diabetes must approach physical participation with a sound understanding of exercise physiology. The successful management of blood glucose levels poses a major challenge for active people with insulin-treated diabetes (and, in some cases, for those who take oral antidiabetic medications). Diabetic athletes must know how the body regulates its metabolic fuels before, during, and after exercise and what effects diabetic complications have on exercise capacity and safety.

In *The Diabetic Athlete*, Sheri Colberg has provided an extremely valuable resource for people with diabetes who participate in competitive or recreational sports. She reviews how energy is produced and used by the body during and after exercise and the key role that insulin and the glucose counterregulatory hormones play in maintaining blood glucose levels within a relatively narrow range in nondiabetic people.

Before the availability of blood glucose monitoring, diabetic athletes relied on symptoms of hypoglycemia, prolonged hyperglycemia, and positive urine tests for glucose and ketones to adjust their insulin and dietary regimens for exercise. Today, the ability to test blood glucose at frequent intervals, the availability of a wide range of insulin preparations, and advanced delivery systems make it possible for well-informed diabetic athletes to manage their blood glucose successfully in most situations. Doing this requires knowledge and ingenuity, which can be gained through reading this book.

In *The Diabetic Athlete*, Colberg has assembled a practical and readable book that is invaluable for all diabetic athletes and health care professionals who treat and manage diabetes. She provides detailed discussions of how blood glucose is normally regulated in response to exercise and the principles through which people with diabetes can manage blood glucose during exercise of varying types, duration, and intensity. The book's personal accounts from athletes with diabetes present a range of experiences to learn from.

Edward S. Horton, MD
VP & Director of Clinical Research
Joslin Diabetes Center
Professor of Medicine, Harvard Medical School

preface

Diabetes treatment has gone through dramatic changes in the past two decades. Previously, exercise was often overlooked as a cornerstone in diabetes treatment because it was difficult to maintain blood sugar levels with the additional variability caused by physical activity, especially for people with type 1 diabetes. However, with the availability and affordability of blood glucose self-monitoring, exercise can be done safely and without fear of severely upsetting a delicate glucose balance.

Diagnosed with diabetes myself at the age of four in what I call the Dark Ages of diabetes (1968), I went through childhood, adolescence, and early adulthood without the benefit of a blood glucose meter. I still participated in a variety of sports and physical activities over the years: swimming, running, racquetball, soccer, tennis, weight training, gymnastics, volleyball, cycling, aerobics, dancing, stair climbing, hiking and backpacking, canoeing, football equipment managing, snowshoeing, cross-country and downhill skiing, horseback riding, sailing, snorkeling, skydiving, and child-rearing! I did many of these things while feeling less than my physical best because I was not able to test my blood sugar; I was often either hyperglycemic or hypoglycemic while doing these activities. While growing up, exercise of any kind made me feel better overall, although at the time I did not understand the physiology behind it enough to know why. I felt I had more control over my diabetes as well. So I began exercising regularly on my own and through team sports as a teenager and have continued exercising throughout my adulthood.

Not until I had a blood glucose meter did I realize, however, how much better I felt during exercise when my blood sugars were in a more normal range. Keeping them normal with the help of a blood glucose meter has totally been a trial-and-error learning process! At the time I got my first meter, there were very few guidelines or books that could offer me any guidance. I did eventually learn to control my blood sugars for various activities, but every time I tried a new or unusual one, it was like starting over again. When I attended my first IDAA (International Diabetic Athletes Association) meeting in Phoenix, Arizona, in 1990, I met a lot of other active people. It struck me then that I could learn so much from others' experiences that could make my trial-and-error process shorter and easier. It was from this experience that I eventually got the idea and motivation for this book.

In 1998 I sent out a questionnaire to all English-speaking members of the IDAA (approximately 1,700 people) and received responses from about 250 members. My questionnaire asked them to describe their usual diets, medications, and exercise routines. Additionally, I asked them to describe the specific alterations in these variables that they make for any of a variety of sports and recreational physical activities. I also asked them to indicate the degree to which they follow current and past exercise guidelines. This book is a compilation of their experiences, and I hope that each of you can use it to attain better blood sugar control while exercising.

Part I of this book covers the basics about exercise. I have always found that knowledge is power when it comes to managing diabetes. I researched information for years, which finally resulted in my earning a doctoral degree in exercise physiology from the University of California at Berkeley. You do not need a PhD to understand how your body adapts to exercise, but you do need to understand the basics in order to make safe changes in your diet and medication.

Chapter 1 deals with the basics of exercise prescription: how to monitor your exercise intensity, what type of exercise to do, how often to exercise, and for how long. If you really want to improve your fitness and endurance, you will benefit from understanding how to work out properly. The intensity determines the overload on your muscles and your subsequent fitness gains. Warm-ups and cooldowns are important for all athletes, but especially for diabetic athletes who may have some unique concerns.

Chapter 2 is key to understanding your blood sugar response to any activity. Once you can determine what energy systems and fuels your body uses during the exercise, then you can virtually predict what your blood sugar response will be and what you need to do to maintain normal sugars during and following the activity. It is also important to understand how circulating insulin alters your normal response to an activity and how chronic training affects fuel utilization.

Chapter 3 will help you understand the types of medications and regimens that people use to either replace insulin or improve its production and action. Again, differing insulin regimens, timing of exercise, and sensitivity to insulin greatly affect your circulating insulin levels. Exercise in the morning can result in a very different response than exercise at another time of day. It is also important that you recognize all the potential symptoms of hypoglycemia, especially if you have not had many episodes and realize that symptoms may be different during exercise and after training.

Chapter 4 addresses some of the nutritional and ergogenic substances currently on the market in terms of their effectiveness and their safety for athletes, specifically diabetic athletes. This chapter is by no means comprehensive, but it does address how nutritional supplements affect athletic performance and blood sugar regulation during exercise. Supplements of potential benefit or harm to diabetic athletes are noted.

Chapters 5 and 6 address some special concerns and precautions for athletes with type 1 and type 2 diabetes, respectively. Chapter 5 specifically relays some of the athletes' responses to published exercise guidelines and gives you the benefit of knowing how other people use these guidelines. Diabetic complications are, unfortunately, a reality for many people with diabetes; you can still exercise, but certain precautions are discussed to make exercise safer.

Part II of this book can really help you reduce your trial-and-error time for almost any conceivable sport or physical activity! It is arranged into four chapters by type of activity: endurance sports including the basic sports like running, swimming, and cycling, as well as training for the avid athlete; power sports including recreational sports like basketball and softball; fitness activities such as aerobics, weight training, and other gym workouts; and finally, recreational sports including the current crazes like rock climbing, in-line skating, and snowboarding. Each chapter gives general recommendations for diet and medication changes for each specific sport or activity as well as real-life examples from diabetic athletes who participate in those sports.

While simple guidelines can never be effective for everyone due to individual variability, you can benefit from the knowledge of others' experiences. It is my belief that this combination of basic (the why of exercise) and experiential (the how of exercise) information can benefit all of us in maintaining blood sugars during any physical endeavor. So lose the excuses! Whether you are interested in just recreating or want to be a serious competitive athlete, it is time to get out there and exercise!

acknowledgments

I would like to acknowledge all the individuals who really helped me to create my book so that I could fulfill my dream of helping others with diabetes enjoy the benefits of exercise in their lives.

I would like to thank Paula Harper, founder and president of the International Diabetic Athletes Association (IDAA), who facilitated sending out my exercise questionnaire to most of the IDAA members. I am also truly thankful to all of the IDAA members and other individuals with diabetes who took the time to fill out my questionnaire and mail it back to me. Without their input, I would have had very few real-life examples to share. I would also like to thank Anne Chisholm, formerly of the ODU Research Foundation, who helped me enhance my questionnaire and expand it so that I got enough usable information to put in a book and some published articles.

I would also like to acknowledge all the hard-working individuals at Human Kinetics who helped to make my book a reality. Martin Barnard helped me immensely in doing the initial rewrites by suggesting elements for the book that would really enhance it. Cassandra Mitchell worked with me diligently to edit, re-edit, modify, and clarify my writing. Wendy McLaughlin helped to create all the tabled information in the last four chapters to make it easier to access. Ginny Davis helped with the marketing and promotion of my book along with Kirk Brauer, who worked on getting out the promotional information for the catalog. Jan Feeney helped by copyediting my book, and Sandra Merz Bott helped me immensely with the index. Countless others worked behind the scenes to make my book one I am proud of. I thank you all.

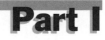

Part I

The Diabetic Athlete's Toolbox

Chapter 1

Training for Sports and Fitness

If you are already an avid exerciser, then you are aware of most of the benefits of exercise for your physical health and your diabetes control. If you are thinking about getting serious about sports or fitness activities, then you have a lot of positive changes to look forward to. In addition to the treats you may be more able to allow yourself after exercising (an ice cream sundae, for example), exercise can help you build muscle and lose body fat, suppress your appetite, eat more without gaining fat weight, enhance your mood, reduce stress and anxiety levels, increase your energy level, improve your immunity, keep your joints and muscles more flexible, and improve the quality of your life!

Physical fitness has undeniable health benefits for all people. Those people who engage in moderate exercise regularly are at lower risk for many chronic health problems including heart disease, obesity, hypertension, type 2 diabetes, certain cancers, and other metabolic disorders. The usual health benefits of exercise apply to people with diabetes as well, perhaps even more so than to people without diabetes. Much of what we attribute to the aging process—muscle atrophy or loss of flexibility in joints—really results from disuse. Diabetes, especially when blood sugar levels are poorly controlled, accelerates the aging process as well as certain disease processes such as heart disease. Thus, regular exercise can slow the aging process and reduce long-term complications associated with diabetes. These benefits cannot be understated! Not only can you enjoy your favorite physical activities, you can also help your health.

Regular exercise is the most important activity you can do to slow the aging process, manage your blood sugars, and reduce your risk of diabetic complications.

Exercise provides additional benefits for people with diabetes:

- Improvements in insulin sensitivity, resulting in less insulin needed to maintain normal blood sugar levels
- Decreased cardiovascular risk factors with increases in HDL-cholesterol and reductions in LDL-cholesterol and circulating triglycerides
- Enhanced fibrinolysis (reduced blood platelet stickiness and less chance for formation of blood clots leading to heart attacks or strokes)
- Improvements in psychological status and coping with stress related to diabetes or other stressors
- Increased muscle mass and reduced body fat, both of which also contribute to improvements in insulin sensitivity
- Potential improvements in overall glycemic control if blood sugars are monitored and adjustments are made in diet and medications

Fitness can be defined many different ways. Most important to overall health is aerobic fitness, or physical conditioning resulting from prolonged aerobic activities such as brisk walking, jogging, cycling, swimming, rowing, and aerobic dance. An aerobic exercise program incorporates all of the following components in determining the level of fitness you achieve: the type of exercise you choose to do (mode), how hard (intensity), how long (duration), how often you exercise (frequency), and your rate of progression. You and your physician or exercise professional should develop an exercise prescription with careful consideration of your health status (diabetes control, complications, and other health problems), risk factors for cardiovascular disease, personal goals, and exercise preferences.

COMPONENTS OF AEROBIC EXERCISE

Even if you are already an avid exerciser, it is still helpful to review this basic information. The American College of Sports Medicine (ACSM) publishes guidelines based on all the current research that address the basics of an individualized exercise prescription with regard to mode of exercise, intensity, duration, frequency, and progression of training. Whether you are already a regular exerciser or just beginning, these basic principles still apply to improving your fitness level and controlling your blood sugar levels.

Mode

The greatest improvements in maximal oxygen consumption ($\dot{V}O_2$max) and endurance occur with exercise involving the large muscle groups continuously performing rhythmic, prolonged activities such as walking, running, swimming, cycling, rowing, in-line skating, and cross-country skiing. Anaerobic strength training is not a usual means to increase $\dot{V}O_2$max, but it is an important component to increase muscular strength and muscular endurance as well as lean body mass. Resistance training (strength training), and other near-maximal exercise can be used as stimuli to prevent the loss of lean muscle mass that normally occurs with aging and disuse. These gains in muscle mass can also increase your daily caloric needs and improve your insulin sensitivity and blood glucose control. However, to achieve optimal cardiovascular fitness, your exercise program must include an aerobic component.

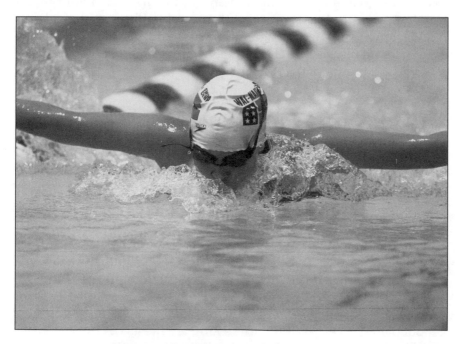

Swimming is an excellent activity to help you achieve optimal cardiovascular fitness and gains in $\dot{V}O_2$max.

Intensity

Your choice of exercise intensity should reflect your training goals (i.e., greater caloric expenditure versus maximal increases in endurance performance or $\dot{V}O_2$max). Intensity and duration of exercise are interrelated. Usually higher-intensity exercises cannot be sustained as long as lower-intensity activities, but the greater overload that the higher-intensity exercise provides leads to more significant improvements in performance. If your goal is weight loss, doing an activity at a lower intensity for longer duration is usually more effective. You should consider your initial fitness level as well as the goals of your exercise, your risks for orthopedic or cardiovascular problems, the presence of diabetes-related complications, and your personal preferences.

Exercise intensity can be monitored in various ways. The ACSM recommends that the exercise intensity be in the range of 60 to 90 percent of your maximum heart rate, or 50 to 85 percent of $\dot{V}O_2$max or heart rate reserve. Heart rate (HR) can be used as a measure of intensity because it is linearly related to oxygen consumption ($\dot{V}O_2$). The goal of exercise is to maintain a heart rate in your target training range for the duration of the exercise. Since maximal heart rate declines linearly with age, it is best if your maximal heart rate can be directly measured. However, it can be estimated fairly accurately using the following formula:

$$\text{Max HR} = 220 - \text{age}$$

For example, a 35-year-old athlete would have an estimated maximal heart rate of 185 beats per minute (220 minus 35). The intensity range is 60 to 90 percent of the actual or estimated maximal heart rate (see table 1.1), a range of 111 to 167 beats per minute for this athlete. Be aware that certain medications such as beta-blockers like Lopressor or Inderal can reduce your rest and exercise heart rates. If you take such medications, expect your estimated maximal and submaximal heart rates to be lower than normal.

You can determine a more accurate and individualized heart rate range using the Karvonen method to calculate your heart rate reserve or HRR (HRR = maximal heart rate minus resting heart rate). It is best to measure your resting heart rate upon waking before you get out of bed. Then multiply this estimated "reserve" by 50 percent and 85 percent before adding it back to your resting heart rate to determine your lower and upper limits (a range of 50 to 85 percent of heart rate reserve).

Table 1.1   **Target Heart Rate (HR) Ranges**

Age	Max HR	60% range	75% range	90% range
20-29	191-200	115-120	143-150	172-180
30-39	181-190	109-114	136-142	163-171
40-49	171-180	103-108	129-135	154-162
50-59	161-170	97-102	121-128	145-153
60-69	151-160	91-96	113-120	136-144

Note: Maximal HR is estimated as 220 minus age in years when actual maximal HR has not been measured.

$$\text{Lower limit HR} = 0.50 \,(\text{max HR} - \text{rest HR}) + \text{rest HR}$$
$$\text{Upper limit HR} = 0.85 \,(\text{max HR} - \text{rest HR}) + \text{rest HR}$$

For example, if our 35-year-old athlete has a resting heart rate of 72, her HRR is 113 beats per minute (185 minus 72). Her range is then 50 to 85 percent of HRR added to her resting value, or a range of 128 to 168 beats per minute. If maximal oxygen consumption ($\dot{V}O_2$max) is directly measured during an exercise test on a treadmill or a cycle ergometer, then the corresponding heart rates for 50 percent and 85 percent can be directly determined from the maximal test and alternately used as the training range. (For a person with a very low fitness level, ACSM recommends exercise with a starting intensity of 40 percent rather than 50 percent.)

Another method to monitor intensity is Borg's Rating of Perceived Exertion (RPE) scale. This scale allows you to subjectively measure how hard you feel you are working (see table 1.2). The recommended range of RPE for optimal fitness improvement is 12 to 16 ("somewhat hard" to "hard") on the category (original) scale with 20 being the very hardest level. On the category ratio scale that ranges from 0 to 20, you should exercise at a level of 4 to 5. Working out below these ranges may not overload your system enough to cause significant adaptive changes, and working above them may limit the duration and aerobic nature of the activity. You can also use the talk test to ensure that your exercise intensity is not too hard: if you are breathing too hard to carry on a conversation with an exercise partner, then your intensity is above the recommended range.

The intensity of exercise is probably the most important factor in improving performance and maintaining your fitness level even with a decrease in frequency or duration of exercise. Pre-event tapers (decreased training volume) are most effective if you maintain the intensity of workouts. With diabetes, although you may effectively

Table 1.2 **Rating of Perceived Exertion (RPE) Scales**

Original Scale		Category Ratio	
6		0	Nothing at all
7	Very, very light	0.5	Very, very weak
8		1	Very weak
9	Very light	2	Weak
10		3	Moderate
11	Fairly light	4	Somewhat strong
12		5	Strong
13	Somewhat hard	6	
14		7	Very strong
15	Hard	8	
16		9	
17	Very hard	10	Very, very strong
18		*	Maximal
19	Very, very hard	Borg RPE Scale © Gunnar Borg,	
20		1970, 1985, 1984, 1998	

maintain your fitness levels during pre-event tapering, you have to be prepared to increase your insulin doses or reduce your food intake during a taper because your overall caloric expenditure will be less. Reduced training volume will also result in less blood glucose and muscle glycogen use. If you decrease your exercise intensity as well, you may need even greater regimen changes to keep blood sugars from rising.

Duration

The ACSM recommends 20 to 60 minutes of continuous aerobic activity to sufficiently improve your fitness level. Although some improvements in endurance have been shown with very intense exercise (more than 90 percent of $\dot{V}O_2$max) lasting only five to 10 minutes, this type of exercise is much more risky for injuries and cardiovascular events. Also, you achieve a greater total caloric expenditure by exercising over a longer duration at a lower, more sustainable intensity. You may also do two or three bouts of shorter exercise during the day (instead of 20 to 60 minutes continuously) and achieve almost the same fitness gain. If you train for an event such as a marathon run, you will need to engage in longer workouts, on occasion longer than the recommended 60 minutes, to prepare for your run, but an athlete training to participate in a 5K run (3.1 miles) may not benefit from longer workouts. Usually increases in duration beyond 60 minutes do not increase fitness gains significantly enough to compensate for the large increases in overuse and other orthopedic injuries resulting from such ultraendurance exercise.

Frequency

Frequency is interrelated with both intensity and duration of exercise. The ACSM recommends exercising a minimum of three to five

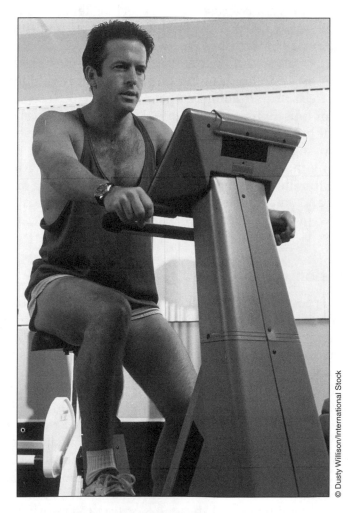

© Dusty Willison/International Stock

Try stationary cycling for a 20-minute minimum or combine cycling with another aerobic conditioning machine to equal a 20-minute workout.

days per week. People with a lower exercise capacity who may not be able to meet the recommended duration of exercise may benefit from more frequent exercise sessions interspersed throughout the day. Athletes who train for a specific event or sport may work out more often in order to optimize their readiness for the event.

Generally, you should exercise almost daily to establish a consistent effect on your blood sugars; however, with blood glucose monitoring and other methods of glycemic control, you can still control your blood sugars if you don't exercise every day. Furthermore, taking at least one day a week to rest allows your body time to recuperate and may prevent overuse injuries such as tendinitis and stress fractures. In any case, you can maintain your current fitness level with a minimum of two days per week of activity.

The ACSM also recommends engaging in resistance-type training as well as flexibility training a minimum of two to three days per week. Resistance training has been shown to be essential to prevent loss of muscle tissue over time. Having more muscle will increase your basal metabolic rate and calorie expenditure every day, thus improving insulin sensitivity and preventing some fat weight gains. Many more older individuals are now engaging in regular resistance training to combat the usual effects of aging and disuse on muscle and bone mass. Flexibility training is also essential in preventing loss of joint mobility (see discussion of this topic later in this chapter).

Progression

The rate of progression for an activity varies on an individual basis. The usual recommended exercise progression consists of an initial conditioning phase lasting four to six weeks, an improvement phase lasting four to five months, and a maintenance phase from six months on. If you already have a high level of fitness, you may shorten or skip the initial stage altogether. During the progression stage, you will make more rapid gains in fitness if you maintain exercise intensity closer to the high end of your recommended ranges (near 90 percent of maximal heart rate or 85 percent of heart rate reserve or $\dot{V}O_2max$). Once in the maintenance stage, you will experience minimal further improvements unless you continue to increase the conditioning stimulus either by increasing intensity, duration, or frequency, or a combination of these. According to the overload principle of training, your muscles and cardiovascular system must

Michelle McGann

"It's the saucy wide-brimmed hats she wears that really have the crowds talking."

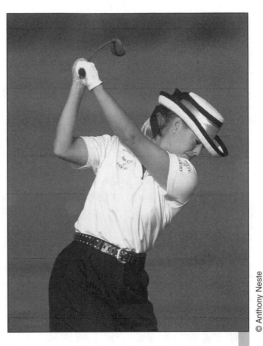

© Anthony Neste

When LPGA Tour professional golfer Michelle McGann steps onto the fairway to play in a tournament, she is immediately recognized by her hats, not by her diabetes. Michelle was bitten by the golfing bug at the age of eight when she first popped a ball onto the fairway. Diagnosed with type 1 diabetes at the age of 13, Michelle never gave up her dream of becoming a pro golfer. She continued playing golf almost daily, and she decided that she was not going to let diabetes handicap her. She qualified for the LPGA in 1989 when she was only 18 years old after an impressive showing in the U.S. Open in 1988, which she entered as an amateur. Her trademark hats came along later in 1991, along with commercial endorsements for designer clothing, a whole line of Michelle McGann jewelry, and other accessories. In addition to her fashion-consciousness, Michelle is capable of making some of the longest drives in women's golf today (often 260 yards or more). With at least seven LPGA titles under her belt, she is certainly a seasoned professional. In 1997, she crossed the $2 million mark in career earnings.

Playing professional golf with diabetes does have its rough spots, though. It involves lengthy tournaments from January to September, endless days of practice, and a lot of environmental extremes like hot and humid days. Michelle says, "I have the ups and downs, of course. At times the adrenaline is really flowing, and it's hard to know how much insulin to take. Other times I know something is wrong because I feel tired and my swing gets weaker. But when you're a professional you have to keep going." She has only had one serious insulin reaction while playing, which occurred during a junior tournament. In those days, she was not allowed to talk with anyone or carry her own bag. She passed out on the fairway before she could tell her parents that her blood sugar was too low. Fortunately, things are much different on the fairways now.

Michelle keeps her diabetes in close control by testing her blood sugar levels and carrying quick sugar sources and snacks in her golf bag. She feels that all of the exercise she gets by golfing actually helps her to control her blood sugars. She also coordinates an annual golf tournament to raise money for diabetes research. Meanwhile, she continues to concentrate on playing golf, improving her game, winning, and having fun with it all.

continue to be appropriately stressed for any further fitness adaptations to occur.

COMPONENTS OF A WORKOUT

Having reviewed what components you need to consider in your exercise program, you also need to consider what comprises each workout. An exercise session should consist of a warm-up, an aerobic exercise, and a cool-down (see figure 1.1). The warm-up and cooldown periods should consist of a similar aerobic activity at a lower intensity, such as slow jogging before and after a faster run. A good warm-up is at least five minutes of an activity before the intensity is increased to meet the ACSM's guidelines to improve aerobic fitness. An appropriate cool-down is five minutes of the same activity after the more intense activity. Your workout session should also include a period of five to ten minutes of static stretching of the major muscle groups. You can stretch before and after exercise. The key is to stretch to the point of discomfort, back off just a little bit, and then hold the stretch at that point for 10 to 30 seconds without bouncing. Bouncing elicits the muscles' stretch reflexes, and you may end up contracting the muscle or muscles you are trying to relax. It is usually easier to stretch once you have warmed up the muscles and joints and increased blood flow to those areas.

It is especially important for people with diabetes to take the time to warm up, cool down, and stretch properly. People with diabetes form more glycosylation end products than people without diabetes; that is, glucose molecules adhere to various structures in the body including cartilage and collagen, causing them to stiffen and lose their usual flexibility. Although all people lose joint and muscular mobility with age, diabetes accelerates the usual loss of flexibility especially when blood sugar levels are higher and greater glycosylation of bodily structures occurs. The result is that people with diabetes are usually more prone to overuse injuries such as tendinitis (inflammation of the tendons connecting muscle to bone) and diabetic frozen shoulder, a condition characterized by limited and painful movement of the shoulder, and it may also take longer for joint injuries to heal properly if injured. Thus, you especially need to take the time to warm up for at least five minutes before your aerobic exercise session, cool down for five minutes, and stretch the major muscle groups involved in your activity.

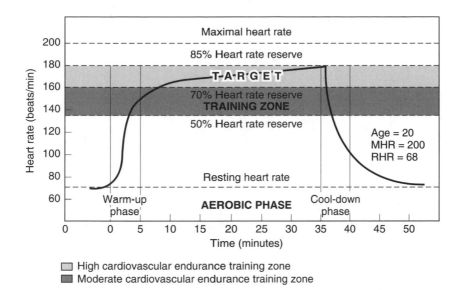

Figure 1.1 Example of an appropriate aerobic workout for a 20-year-old individual with a resting heart rate of 68 beats per minute.

Diabetic people are at higher risk for heart disease and silent heart attacks, and proper warm-ups and cool-downs can help prevent cardiac arrhythmias (abnormal heartbeats) or sudden cardiac events during and following exercise. A proper cool-down is also important as well to prevent blood from pooling in your extremities. People with diabetes are more prone to dehydration when blood sugars run above normal, especially while exercising in a hot environment. The reduced blood volume resulting from a combination of sweating and preexisting dehydration can cause fainting if you stop exercising abruptly without cooling down and allowing your body to redirect blood flow away from your muscles and back to your central circulation.

Following these guidelines can assist you in creating optimal workouts and the most beneficial exercise training program possible. The rewards of your regular workouts will far outweigh any potential problems with managing your diabetes with exercise as a confounding variable.

Chapter 2

Balancing Exercise Blood Sugars

As all people with diabetes know, it is a constant balancing act to keep blood sugars in a normal range. The challenge of doing so with exercise added into the balancing act can feel overwhelming at times. Exercise presents its own special set of problems for control. On the one hand, exercise-induced blood glucose uptake by working muscles may result in hypoglycemia (low blood sugar) during or following exercise. If circulating insulin levels are high at the start of exercise, the extra insulin may cause excessive uptake of glucose during exercise, which results in an episode of hypoglycemia as well. On the other hand, exercising with high blood sugar and ketones (indicating a relative lack of insulin in your body) can cause blood sugars to go even higher, which increases the risk of diabetic ketoacidosis (DKA), which can be life-threatening and require hospitalization. An additional challenge is the risk of postexercise late-onset hypoglycemia, which can occur up to 48 hours following exercise while insulin sensitivity is heightened during the restoration of depleted muscle glycogen (the storage form of glucose in skeletal muscle).

The following are some of the many variables that affect your blood sugar response to exercise: the time of day you exercise; the timing of insulin doses and the types of insulin you use; your insulin injection site; the time you last ate and the type of food you ate; your blood sugar levels when you begin exercising; the type, duration, and intensity of your exercise and how accustomed you are to doing it (training effect); the environmental temperature and conditions; illness; the timing of a woman's menstrual cycle; pregnancy; and your level of hydration.

The best way to deal with the multitude of variables is to learn your own responses to all of them by checking blood sugar levels before, during, and after exercise.

Hopefully, a somewhat predictable pattern will emerge to help you anticipate your responses to future bouts of similar exercise.

ENERGY SYSTEMS AND ATP PRODUCTION

The way energy is used during physical activity affects blood sugar levels. How fast you move, how much force you produce, and how long the activity continues affect the overall energy needs of your working muscles. To deal with these different effects, your body has three distinct energy systems to supply your muscles with ATP (adenosine triphosphate), a high-energy compound found in all cells. ATP is the direct, immediate source of energy for all muscular contractions. Once a nerve impulse initiates a muscle contraction, calcium is released within the muscle cell, ATP "energizes" the muscle fibers, and a muscle contraction occurs. Without ATP, your muscles would not be able to contract. Muscle contains only small quantities of ATP ready for use, enough to fuel any activity for about a second. For an activity to last longer, more ATP must be supplied to the muscle by one or more of the energy systems in your body. For more rapid or more forceful movements, your body must supply ATP at a faster rate. While all the energy systems can supply additional ATP, the rate they can supply it varies. The fuels used to make the ATP and the amount of time needed to supply it also differ according to the energy system. Due to these differences in the fuels used by the energy systems, the type of exercise that you choose to do can affect your blood sugar response differently as well.

ATP-CP System

All muscular contractions are fueled directly by the breakdown of ATP (see figure 2.1). As the force and frequency of contractions in-

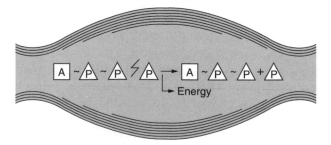

Figure 2.1 ATP directly provides all energy for muscular contractions by removing its last high-energy phosphate group.

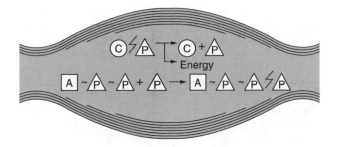

Figure 2.2 Creatine phosphate (CP) provides energy to rapidly replenish ATP during 6 to 8 seconds of all out effort.

crease, the rate of ATP utilization also increases. For very short and powerful activities, one energy system is primarily used to provide the ATP. This phosphagen system, consisting of ATP stored in muscle and crea-tine phosphate (CP), which replenishes ATP, requires no oxygen for energy production and is, therefore, classified as anaerobic in nature (see figure 2.2). Creatine phosphate cannot fuel an activity directly, but the energy released from its rapid breakdown is immediately used to resynthesize ATP for an additional 5 to 10 seconds following the depletion of the initial supply of ATP. Phosphagen stores (ATP and CP) can only fuel an all-out effort for 6 to 8 seconds before being depleted. Thus, any activity lasting 10 seconds or less is fueled mainly by these stored phosphagens in the muscle fibers; these activities include powerlifting, 40-meter sprints, pole vaulting, long jump, pitching, and dunking a basketball. The second energy system (lactic acid system) supplies the additional energy if the activity lasts longer. Generally, these types of activities do not reduce blood sugar levels because glucose is not involved in energy production. Such intense activities can actually raise the blood sugar when accompanied by a heightened release of certain hormones. This effect will be discussed later in this chapter.

Lactic Acid System

Activities lasting longer than 20 seconds and up to two minutes still mainly depend on anaerobic energy produced through a combination of the phosphagens initially and then the breakdown of muscle glycogen, a storage form for glucose in the muscle. This breakdown is called glycogenolysis. Once released from its storage form, energy is produced through the metabolic pathway of glycolysis, which forms lactic acid as a by-product of this rapid anaerobic production of ATP. While glycolysis occurs in the cells under normal resting

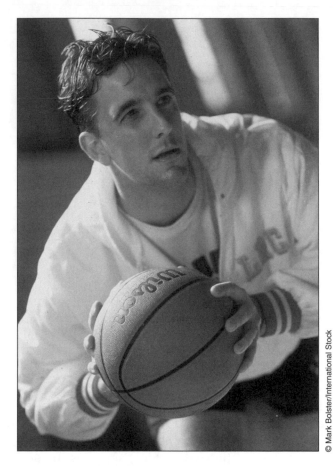

Phosphagen stores (ATP and CP) in muscle provide the energy for you to shoot a basketball.

conditions, the muscles' use of ATP is relatively low and does not result in lactic acid accumulation because glucose and glycogen are processed through aerobic means (using oxygen). See figure 2.3.

With the additional demand for rapid energy when exercise begins, glycolysis proceeds more rapidly to provide more ATP and the system soon becomes limited by the accumulation of lactic acid. When large quantities are present in muscle, lactic acid drops the pH of muscle and blood, causing the "burn" you feel in those muscles and adversely affecting your ability to continue. Only three ATP are produced from each glucosyl unit released from muscle glycogen, which is a relatively small amount compared with ATP production through aerobic means. Consequently, this system cannot supply enough energy for prolonged periods of exercise. Activities that pri-

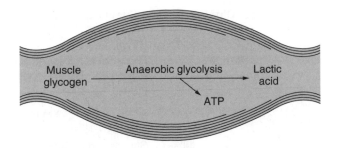

Figure 2.3 The breakdown of muscle glycogen through glycolysis results in ATP and lactic acid production and provides energy for activities lasting 20 seconds to two minutes.

marily depend on this energy system include 800-meter runs, 200-meter swimming events, and stop-and-start activities like basketball, lacrosse, field hockey, and ice hockey.

Studies of people with type 1 and type 2 diabetes have shown that very intense exercise such as resistance training, weightlifting, or near-maximal aerobic exercise can actually cause an immediate rise in blood sugar levels due to the body's hormonal response to the workload. Intense exercise causes the release of several hormones in the body that increase the liver's production of glucose and reduce the muscles' uptake of blood sugar. These hormones include epinephrine (adrenaline) and norepinephrine, which are released by the sympathetic nervous system in response to intense exercise, as well as glucagon, growth hormone, and cortisol (see table 2.1). The effects of these counterregulatory (glucose-raising) hormones can easily exceed your body's immediate need for and use of glucose, especially because exercise at such a high intensity cannot be sustained for very long. The result of this "feedforward" hormonal control of blood glucose production is a rise in blood sugar during and following intense exercise.

Intense exercise can cause a large increase in blood sugars due to the surge in glucose-raising hormones.

A state of insulin resistance is induced, which can last for a few hours after exercise. After doing near-maximal cycling to exhaustion, one group of people with type 1 diabetes on insulin pumps was found to have an elevated blood glucose level for two hours following this activity. Additional insulin is needed to bring blood sugar levels back to normal following such intensive exercise. A similar rise in blood glucose levels for a group of people with type 2

Table 2.1 **Hormones With Glucose-Raising Effects During Exercise**

Hormone	Source	Main actions during exercise
Glucagon	Pancreas	Stimulation of liver glycogen breakdown and new glucose production from precursors to increase glucose output; large effect of changes in the insulin-to-glucagon ratio
Epinephrine	Adrenal medulla	Stimulation of muscle and, to a lesser extent, liver, glycogen breakdown, and mobilization of free fatty acids from adipose (fat) tissues
Norepinephrine	Adrenal medulla, sympathetic nerve endings	Stimulation of liver to produce new glucose from available precursors; "feedforward" control of glucose during intense exercise along with epinephrine
Growth hormone	Anterior pituitary	Direct stimulation of fat metabolism (release of free fatty acids from adipose) and indirect suppression of glucose use; stimulation of amino acid storage
Cortisol	Adrenal cortex	Mobilization of amino acids and glycerol as precursors for glucose production by the liver and release of free fatty acids for muscle use in lieu of glucose

diabetes was evident for one hour after maximal cycling exercise, along with large increases in circulating insulin levels. An increase in insulin following intensive exercise is also normally found in people without diabetes. However, once these hormonal effects wane, increased rates of glycogen repletion can cause your blood sugars to decrease more later on, potentially resulting in hypoglycemia.

Aerobic System

The other end of the energy system spectrum is the aerobic energy system used for prolonged, endurance, or ultraendurance exercise. Due to their duration, these activities mainly depend on aerobic production of energy (the oxygen system). Your muscles must have a steady supply of ATP to be active during sustained physical activity. Aerobic activities such as walking, running, swimming, cycling, rowing, and cross-country skiing, are done continuously for longer than two minutes. Running a marathon or ultramarathon, doing a full-length triathlon, or participating in subsequent full days of endurance exercise such as long-distance cycling, walking, running, or backpacking are more extreme examples of prolonged aerobic activities.

The fuels for these aerobic activities are mainly a mix of carbohydrate and fat. Protein can be used to fuel an activity, but they are usually metabolized during very prolonged endurance activities such as running a marathon, and then only to a minor extent (providing less than 10 percent of the total energy). At rest, your diet affects the mix of fuels your body uses, but most people generally use a mix of about 60 percent fat and 40 percent carbohydrate. Carbohydrate utilization increases rapidly when you begin to exercise and increases with any additional increment in exercise intensity. High-intensity or near-maximal activities use 100 percent carbohydrate and zero percent fat during the activity. Muscle glycogen is used most during this intensity of exercise, along with blood glucose. Circulating hormones such as epinephrine mobilize fats from adipose stores (mostly subcutaneous depots below the skin), which circulate in the blood as free fatty acids that active muscles use during less intense activities (see figure 2.4). This fat source and some intramuscular stores are used more extensively during mild to moderate activities along with some carbohydrate. During recovery from exercise, the predominant fuel source is again fat—this time derived mainly from intramuscular triglyceride stores.

Thus, both anaerobic energy systems (the phosphagens and the lactic acid system) are important at the beginning of any longer-duration

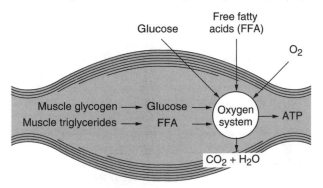

Figure 2.4 The aerobic system supplies ATP for longer-duration activities from blood and intramuscular carbohydrate and fat sources.

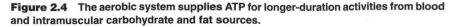

exercise before aerobic metabolism supplies enough ATP (see figure 2.5). The anaerobic systems are also important when the intensity of a prolonged activity increases (for example, beginning to run uphill or sprinting to the finish line of a 10K race). The actual aerobic fuels your body uses during the activity, however, depend on your training status, your diet before and during the activity, the intensity and duration of the activity, and your circulating levels of insulin during the activity.

TRAINING EFFECTS ON FUEL USE

Training improves your body's capacity to metabolize fat, which results in a greater use of fat, a slower depletion of muscle glycogen, and a reduced use of blood glucose during an activity once your muscles have adapted to it by doing your training regimen. The training effect on fuel utilization is very evident in people with diabetes. It manifests as an eventual reduced need for additional carbohydrate during an activity after doing the same activity for several weeks. Chronic exercise training has been shown to decrease the hormonal response to submaximal exercise. When a diabetic athlete follows a training regimen, less of the glucose-raising hormones are

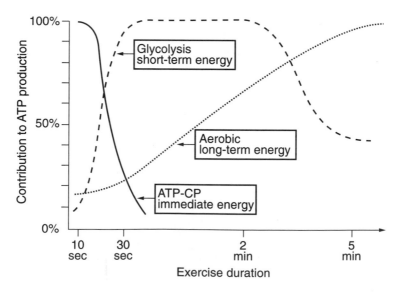

Figure 2.5 Exercise duration largely determines the overall contribution of the three energy systems during an activity.

released in response to exercise of the same intensity (i.e., less glucagon, epinephrine, norepinephrine, growth hormone, and cortisol are released). In a nondiabetic person, a smaller reduction in insulin in response to exercise also occurs. The result of all these differences is a reduced use of blood glucose and muscle glycogen and a greater use of fat for the same intensity of exercise after training—all of which result in more normal (higher) blood sugar levels (less risk of hypoglycemia) during the activity. This change in fuel use explains why diabetic people need to eat more carbohydrates to maintain blood sugar levels when initially participating in an activity; but they need to eat less for the same activity after doing it for several weeks.

You may find that after training for several weeks, your blood glucose does not drop as significantly as it did when you first started training.

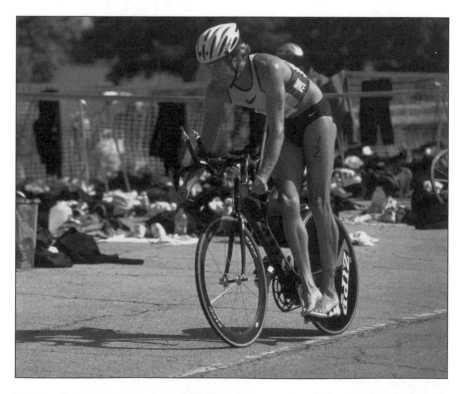

Participation in triathlons uses a significant amount of carbohydrate mainly through the use of muscle glycogen and blood glucose.

If you increase the intensity of an activity after training to maintain the same relative level of work, however, your carbohydrate use during the activity may be just as high as before the training. This effect is also sport-specific, which means that if your training consists of running, your blood sugars probably will not be maintained equally well if you start swimming laps but have not done any swim training.

CARBOHYDRATE USE

During prolonged aerobic activities that require a substantial amount of carbohydrate to fuel the activity, starting with adequate muscle glycogen stores is critical in preventing fatigue. During aerobic activities that are sustained for 60 to 90 minutes, fatigue may be related to total muscle glycogen depletion or depletion within specific muscle fibers that you are using (more likely the faster-twitch fibers during higher-intensity activities). For longer but lower-intensity activities, your body more readily uses blood glucose along with muscle glycogen. In those cases when fatigue occurs after 90 minutes or longer, the likely cause is general depletion of carbohydrate stores in the body. This includes a depletion of muscle glycogen as well as liver glycogen, which may lead to hypoglycemia. When you ingest carbohydrate during exercise, you can delay the decline in blood glucose and you can sustain exercise for a longer period of time. People with diabetes should prevent hypoglycemic fatigue by making regimen changes, which include reduced insulin doses and increased carbohydrate intake.

In general, carbohydrate is recommended during exercise due to its rapid metabolism and absorption compared to fat and protein. The amount and type of carbohydrates (simple versus complex) may depend on factors such as the duration of the exercise and its intensity, your blood sugar levels before and during the exercise, the time of day that you exercise, and whether injected insulins are peaking.

The type of carbohydrate you ingest can affect your blood sugar response. One research study measured blood sugar levels in fasting, exercising diabetic people in response to ingestion of glucose, white bread, or nothing. The exercise consisted of 45 minutes of riding a cycle ergometer at a moderate intensity (60 percent of $\dot{V}O_2max$) in the morning before injecting any insulin. Without any carbohydrate, blood sugar levels fell slightly in these people despite having the

Chris Dudley

"Banging, battling, and pounding, he earns his living the hard way— as an NBA center."

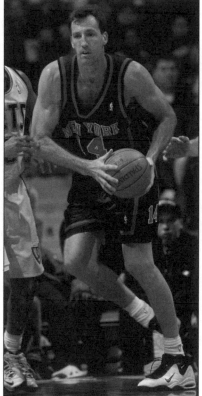

© Ezra O. Shaw/Allsport

An inch shy of seven feet tall, Chris Dudley was a low pick in the NBA draft (75th) in 1987, but he has nevertheless made quite a name for himself in the professional ranks playing center for a number of pro teams including the Cleveland Cavaliers, the New Jersey Nets, the Portland Trail Blazers, and currently the New York Knicks, where he has played since 1997. He usually plays the crucial role of defender and rebounder for the team, with over 5,100 career rebounds to date. Chris had humble beginnings in the sport playing basketball in his early years one-on-one with his father. In those days, he was still short and anything but a star player. Even in high school, he was often only a benchwarmer fighting to make the varsity team. By his senior year, though, he had become a star player and elected to attend Yale University like his father and grandfather before him. He went on to become a three-time all-Ivy League selection, leading his team in scoring and rebounding in his last two years.

It was during his sophomore year of high school that Chris began to exhibit the classic symptoms of type 1 diabetes. He was thirsty and exhausted all the time. His father recognized the symptoms, tested his urine for sugar, and rushed him to the hospital. Fortunately for him, he was not discouraged from playing the game he loved; the doctors assured him that he could continue to play ball as long as he took care of himself. Playing pro basketball is definitely a challenge, and he knows he has to stay on top of his diabetes with careful planning and preparation to perform well. In addition to testing his blood sugars frequently, he alternates several different daily regimens based on whether it is a game day, a practice day, or a travel day. On game days, he reduces his insulin based on when he is going to exercise intensely, and he checks his sugars before and after the game as well as during half time. He has also worked with a nutritionist and knows which foods to eat for games and travel.

Some of Chris's most crucial contributions are not to basketball, however, but to kids with diabetes. He volunteers his time with the American Diabetes Association and its events such as Walktoberfest. He tells kids, "You can do everything that everybody else does, you just have to be more disciplined." And he practices what he preaches.

lowest levels of circulating insulin in the morning. However, intake of a recommended dose of carbohydrate (30 grams), either as a simple or a complex source, resulted in an excessive rise in blood sugar levels in the majority of these people. Glucose ingestion resulted in almost twice the increase in blood sugar levels as the ingestion of white bread due to differences in their glycemic index, which refers to the rate of absorption into the system and the amount of increase in blood glucose levels that the carbohydrates cause (refer to chapter 4). Thus, it is important for you to monitor and learn your response to exercise with carbohydrate supplementation in order to ascertain the appropriate amount and type of carbohydrate to ingest.

The time of day that you exercise may also play a big role in your need for carbohydrate supplementation. The risk of exercise-induced hypoglycemia is lowest before breakfast, especially if you exercise before any insulin injection. At this time of day, you will generally have lower circulating levels of insulin as well as higher levels of cortisol (a hormone that increases insulin resistance) compared with later in the day. If you exercise following breakfast and an insulin injection, your insulin dose may affect the results. In one study, people with type 1 diabetes performed 60 minutes of moderate cycling starting 90 minutes after administration of regular insulin and breakfast. To prevent hypoglycemia in these insulin pump users, their short-acting insulin bolus was reduced by 50 percent and their basal insulin was discontinued during the activity. Compared with exercise later in the day, though, the morning insulin reductions were still less than afternoon exercise would require.

You are likely to need less supplemental carbohydrate when you exercise early in the morning or when your circulating insulin levels are lower.

INSULIN LEVELS AND EXERCISE

The degree of insulinization (circulating levels of insulin) before and during exercise in people with diabetes is also critical to exercise performance and prevention of fatigue. In nondiabetic people, the concomitant fall in insulin and rise in glucagon are the major determinants of glucose production by the liver during moderate exercise. An excess of insulin during exercise increases blood glucose uptake additively with muscle contractions while reducing the availability of free fatty acids, resulting in hypoglycemia. Hyperglycemia (high blood sugar) during exercise can have a mass action effect, causing a somewhat greater use of blood glucose (and lesser use of muscle glycogen) during an activity.

Your body needs a certain amount of circulating insulin available during exercise. Too little circulating insulin during an activity can lead to an excessive hormonal response that may elevate blood glucose levels and ketone body production. On the other hand, if circulating insulin levels are high during an activity, those levels may inhibit the release of some of the glucose-raising hormones and their effects. The effects of epinephrine are to mobilize fat stores and cause muscle glycogen breakdown, while glucagon increases glucose production by the liver. Without the usual actions of these hormones, your rate of blood glucose uptake into muscle can exceed your liver's glucose production, resulting in hypoglycemia. Refer to figure 2.6.

Exercise is one of the main causes of hypoglycemia in people with tightly controlled diabetes. In one study, intense, exhaustive cycling with too little circulating insulin resulted in hyperglycemia and exaggerated lipolysis (mobilization of fats), while the same exercise with too much insulin resulted in hypoglycemia and a reduced release of fats. While some insulin must be available for a normal metabolic response, exercising with low levels of circulating insulin is indeed a much more normal physiological response. Blood glucose is still taken up by active muscle by contraction-induced mechanisms (not involving insulin) during exercise, but at least with the lower insulin levels, it is not taken up additively by both the actions of insulin and contractions in muscle.

Plasma insulin level during exercise	Liver glucose production	Muscle glucose uptake	Blood glucose
Normal exercise level	⇧	⇧	→
Markedly decreased	⇧	↑	↑
Above normal	↑	⇧	↓

Figure 2.6 Your blood glucose response to exercise is greatly affected by circulating plasma insulin levels, which can alter liver production and muscle uptake of blood sugar.

Circulating insulin levels between exercise sessions can also affect your subsequent exercise performance. In people with diabetes, less muscle glycogen may be stored before or restored after exercise when insulin levels are insufficient or insulin resistance is higher. Although muscle glycogen resynthesis occurs without insulin for the first hour following depleting exercise, glucose uptake after an hour (and your resulting glycogen storage) depends on the presence of sufficient circulating levels of insulin and appropriate insulin action. If less glycogen is stored as a result of insufficient insulin or a high degree of insulin resistance, a higher rate of fat oxidation during lower-intensity exercise may have to compensate for the decreased availability of muscle glycogen. If more blood glucose has to be used during higher-intensity exercise as a result of less glycogen being available for use, fatigue from muscle glycogen depletion or low circulating glucose levels may occur at an earlier time during the activity.

EXERCISE EFFECTS ON INSULIN SENSITIVITY

Physically trained people with diabetes have a heightened sensitivity to insulin, which allows glucose to enter the muscle more efficiently, both acutely and chronically with exercise.

Regular physical activity improves blood glucose control by increasing the body's sensitivity to insulin.

This effect is especially evident in people with type 2 diabetes who are most resistant to insulin. Acute changes in insulin action result from an increased rate of muscle glycogen repletion, whereas chronic changes may be more reflective of increases in the total amount of metabolically active muscle tissue you have. Improvements in insulin action following exercise occur in all people with or without diabetes.

Training adaptations may result in lower insulin needs overall, both basally and specifically for food intake. Reducing your basal levels of insulin as well as your insulin doses for meals before exercise can decrease your risk of hypoglycemia during the activity. An alternative strategy is to exercise when insulin levels are declining or lower, similar to exercise conditions in a nondiabetic person. Many

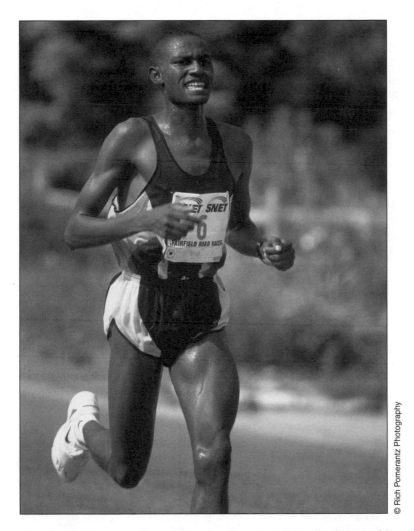

© Rich Pomerantz Photography

Normal training adaptations to marathon running occur in both athletes with well-controlled diabetes, as well as nondiabetic athletes.

people with diabetes prefer to exercise when circulating levels of insulin are low or minimal (at least three to four hours after the last injection of a short-acting insulin) to avoid hypoglycemia.

People with diabetes are probably more aware of the immediate changes in insulin sensitivity than the average person; they notice that they usually need less insulin to eat after an activity. Increases in insulin sensitivity persist after exercise as well, especially during the insulin-independent phase of glycogen repletion (for at least 30 minutes after exercise). This effect may cause hypoglycemia well after exercise has ended. Insulin sensitivity begins to decline after a period of time with no exercise, even in as little as one to two days, despite long-term physical activity. Many athletes report that their total insulin requirements increase after two to three days without their regular exercise.

As previously mentioned, exercise usually positively affects insulin sensitivity, and people with diabetes show an increased sensitivity to insulin shortly after moderate-intensity exercise and even the day after intense exercise. However, one study of type 1 diabetic runners found surprising results: there was no change in insulin sensitivity following a marathon instead of the increased sensitivity found following cross-country skiing. In spite of 50 percent glycogen depletion in these athletes, they were no more insulin sensitive on the day after the marathon than they were on a resting day before the marathon, and they had increased utilization of fats as a fuel. However, these findings were similar to those in nondiabetic people after a marathon. This being the case, this study shows that well-trained diabetic people have enhanced fat utilization and reduced glucose oxidation resulting in the sparing of both blood glucose and muscle glycogen during and after a marathon, similar to nondiabetic people. It appears that this normal training adaptation occurs in people with well-controlled diabetes as well as nondiabetic athletes.

As you can see, many different factors can affect your blood sugar control during and after a workout. Keep in mind that you will tend to lower your blood sugars more when participating in a new or unusual activity, but the intensity and duration of your exercise will also affect glucose use. Intense activities may temporarily raise your blood sugar levels but can cause them to fall later on when the muscle glycogen is being restored. The reward of exercise training, though, is that you will lower your overall insulin needs with regular workouts of any type.

Chapter 3

The Ups and Downs of Insulin

As discussed in chapter 2, when a physical activity begins, a non-diabetic person's body normally shuts down production of insulin and increases the release of glucose-raising (counterregulatory) hormones designed to maintain blood sugar levels in a normal range throughout exercise. For people with diabetes who depend on insulin injections or oral hypoglycemic medications, these normal responses may be altered. It is not possible to "turn off" insulin from an injection site, and in fact, exercise increases blood flow to the muscles and skin, which generally increases the rate of absorption of insulin from these sites. Instead of having less circulating insulin during exercise, you may actually have more than normal, which results in a drop in your blood sugar level. Oral agents can also augment the effects of circulating insulin during exercise or cause a greater insulin release, which results in hypoglycemia.

Circulating levels of insulin greatly affect the blood glucose response to exercise in diabetic people (refer to figure 2.6 in chapter 2). Predicting your response to a given exercise session requires you to take into account the types of insulin you use (shorter-acting and longer-acting insulins have different peak action times and durations), when you injected it, and how much circulating insulin is available before and during any exercise. If you take oral agents, knowing the potential glucose-reducing effects of your medication is important as well.

INSULIN USE

Have you ever just felt like jumping on your bike and going for a ride without giving any thought to where you are going or how long you will be gone? As a person with diabetes, the problem with such spontaneity is that your use of different types of insulin (or oral medications) can affect your circulating levels of insulin during an activity and your ensuing blood sugar response. Different insulins have different times of peak action as well as differing durations, which can make activities, especially spontaneous ones, more problematic. Various insulins are on the market and are used in varying combinations. In general, insulins are considered short-acting, intermediate-acting, or long-acting depending on the onset, peak, and duration of their actions (see table 3.1). Each type of insulin has a different effect on your blood sugar response to exercise. A fact of life for insulin users is that spontaneity must usually be moderated with carbohydrate supplementation or insulin changes to prevent hypoglycemia.

It is crucial to know when your insulins peak in order to determine your blood sugar response to exercise and your need for supplemental carbohydrates.

Of the shorter-acting insulins, human-synthetic Regular insulin is available, but manufacturers have recently discontinued their production of beef and pork combinations. Insulins of synthetic origin in general have faster onset, quicker peak times, and shorter duration than their previous animal counterparts. The latest short-acting insulin to hit the market is Lilly's Humalog (formerly LysPro), which is a very rapid-acting insulin analogue available only with a doctor's prescription. The benefit of Humalog is its short duration: it allows for exercise even two hours following its injection with the lowest risk of insulin-induced hypoglycemia during the activity. Insulin pump users generally use either Humalog, Regular, or a mix of the two insulins in their pumps.

Table 3.1 **Human Insulin Action Times**

Type of insulin	Onset (hr)	Peak (hr)	Duration (hr)	Max duration (hr)
Humalog	<15 min	0.5 – 1.5	2 – 4	4 – 6
Regular	0.5 – 1	2 – 3	3 – 6	6 – 10
NPH	2 – 4	4 – 10	10 – 16	14 – 18
Lente	3 – 4	4 – 12	12 – 18	16 – 20
Ultralente	6 – 10	18 (minimal)	18 – 20	20 – 24

Note: Individual action times may vary depending on a number of factors including environmental conditions, activity level, and injection site.

Many intermediate-acting insulins are available as well. NPH and Lente are the most common insulins of this type. While other intermediate insulins are available, they all generally have the same or similar actions as these two insulins in terms of their onset, peak action, and duration. While some people with type 2 diabetes may use these intermediate insulins alone or a 70/30 mixture of NPH and Regular, most people who use them employ a combination of short- and intermediate-acting insulins throughout the day. A usual regimen is NPH or Lente at breakfast along with Regular or Humalog, with an optional short-acting injection at lunch, a mandatory injection at dinner, and a dose of NPH or Lente at bedtime. An alternate regimen is short-acting insulin doses during the day with a single bedtime dose of NPH or Lente. Clinical research trials are currently being conducted on an insulin called Glargine, an intermediate-acting human synthetic insulin analogue being tested for use as an alternate to NPH, Lente, and Ultralente. NPH and Lente have distinct insulin peaks that can cause hypoglycemia, while Ultralente is notorious for its inconsistent absorption. Studies have shown that Glargine taken in place of NPH doses (on a unit-per-unit basis) resulted in fewer hypoglycemic episodes and effectively provided basal insulin coverage. Some people use NPH in the morning and Lente at bedtime, Lente in the morning and NPH at bedtime, or a combination of these insulins with Ultralente.

Of the longer-acting insulins, the most common is Ultralente. This insulin has a very long duration and a minimal peak. The benefit of Ultralente is that you can fairly effectively replace basal insulin needs with it alone and cover meals and snacks solely with regular or Humalog injections. The difficulty with Ultralente is that changes in its dosage take quite a while to come into effect (often 24-48 hours), and it can be harder to correct in the short term for unusual or prolonged activities with insulin changes alone. Also, as mentioned, its absorption can be inconsistent (due to injection site, activity level, massage, hot tub, or other factors), resulting in basal insulin levels that are too high and then too low.

ORAL MEDICATIONS

It is also important for users of oral hypoglycemic agents to know the general effects of their medications. Oral agents target one or more of three metabolic disorders found in type 2 diabetes: decreased insulin production by the beta cells of the pancreas, elevations in liver production of glucose, or increased insulin resistance in muscle and fat tissues.

Most of the oral agents available are either first- or second-generation medications with differing actions and side effects according to their classification. The first-generation sulfonylureas (i.e., those marketed as Orinase, Dymelor, Tolinase, and Diabinese) generally increase insulin release from the pancreas and decrease insulin resistance. All of the first-generation brands carry a higher risk of interaction with other medications. Diabinese differs the most in its duration of action and side effects because it has the longest duration of the four (up to 72 hours). The other three differ from each other slightly but have a general duration of only 10 to 12 hours. For this reason, Diabinese use carries the greatest risk of hypoglycemia with exercise, especially in patients with kidney dysfunction, because it is not completely metabolized and can accumulate in the body.

Second-generation sulfonylureas include Glucotrol, DiaBeta, Micronase, and Amaryl. Of these four, DiaBeta and Micronase are more likely to cause hypoglycemia during exercise because they have a longer duration of action (24 hours versus 12 to 16 for the other two). In many cases where blood sugars fail to respond to a single oral agent, combination therapies (employing two or more oral agents) are initiated. Such combinations can make the prediction of an exercise response more difficult.

In general, all oral agents with the longest duration, such as Diabinese, DiaBeta, and Micronase, have the greatest potential to cause hypoglycemia during and following exercise, especially when you do an unusual or prolonged activity. New oral drugs hit the market on a daily basis. Many of these drugs attempt to control blood sugars through other physiological avenues. Some recent drugs (a class of drugs called thiazolidinediones) directly enhance peripheral insulin sensitivity without affecting insulin secretion from the pancreas. These are Rezulin, Avandia, and Actos. While hypoglycemia does not typically occur with their use, Rezulin was recently withdrawn from the market due to potential liver damage. Glucophage (metformin) is in a separate class of drugs called biguanides. Its most important action is to reduce the liver's output of glucose, so it can be used in conjunction with other oral medications. In doing so, it is not likely to cause hypoglycemia. Acarbose is an alpha-glucosidase inhibitor used by some people to prevent increases in blood sugar following meals by delaying carbohydrate digestion in the small intestine. In fact, Acarbose is currently being investigated in women with gestational diabetes (during the third trimester of pregnancy). Taking Acarbose before exercise when extra carbohydrate is eaten during exercise could, however, slow the treatment of low blood sugars during exercise. Most of these drugs are used in combination with the oral hypoglycemic agents. However, conversion to insulin therapy is usually necessary when one

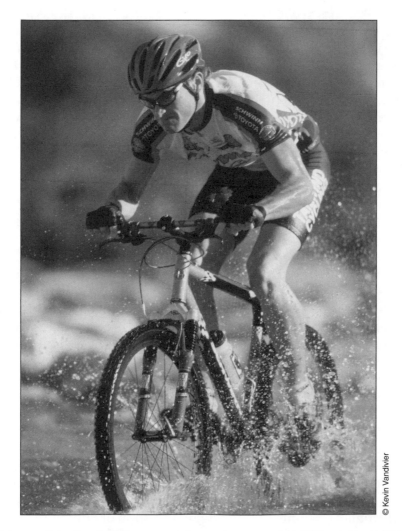

© Kevin Vandivier

Athletes participating in vigorous exercise such as mountain biking may need fairly substantial insulin and dietary regimen changes to compensate.

or more combinations of oral agents as well as the use of these new classes of drugs have failed to control a person's blood sugars.

REGIMEN CHANGES FOR EXERCISE

In part II of this book, recommendations and real-life examples of alterations in insulin and dietary regimens are grouped by basic insulin regimens: pump users, NPH or Lente users, and Ultralente users. *While users of oral hypoglycemic agents are not listed separately, the general recommendations under diet changes alone (or diet changes alone for NPH/Lente users, if the section is divided out) can be used as an approximate guide for these people, especially when blood sugars at the start of or during exercise are in a low to normal range.* As noted previously, certain oral medications carry a higher risk for hypoglycemia and may require more stringent changes in food intake. However, when users of oral agents have elevated preactivity blood sugars, the requisite increases in food intake will be minimal or none. When you start a regular exercise program, monitor your blood sugars frequently to detect any overall changes. Reductions in oral doses of hypoglycemic medications with more regular participation in physical activities may be necessary regardless of the particular medication you use, but you should consult your physician about making any changes once you establish your exercise routine.

While NPH and Lente insulin are grouped together as intermediate-acting insulins, a person's NPH or Lente regimen can vary widely: some users take short-acting insulins (Regular or Humalog) during the day for meals and NPH or Lente at bedtime only, whereas other people take NPH or Lente in both the morning and the evening and even with lunch, resulting in different insulin peaks during the day. You must determine and account for these differences in insulin use depending on your actual insulin regimen.

In many instances, the exercise responses of Ultralente and insulin pump users are more similar as both regimens attempt to provide basal insulin levels. Ultralente has much less of a peak than NPH or Lente and lasts 24 to 48 hours; accordingly, it is intended to provide basal insulin coverage only. Short-acting insulins are administered to cover food intake. Pump users get a continuous infusion of small amounts of either Regular insulin or Humalog to cover basal insulin needs and then supplement with larger boluses of insulin for meals and snacks. In other cases, though, pump users can alter their regimens much differently than Ultralente users due to their ability to suspend the pump and immediately reduce basal rates of insulin.

To confound variables more, some people take a mixture of Regular and Humalog for meals, hoping to cover the later metabolism of proteins and fats more effectively than with Humalog alone, since its actions are so short-lived. For people who take Ultralente during the day (along with short-acting injections for meals and snacks) and NPH or Lente at night, regimen changes are categorized by the insulin that is primarily in effect during exercise.

INSULIN ABSORPTION AND EXERCISE

Exercise, as well as other activities like hot-tubbing or vigorous massage, can increase the absorption rate of injected insulin regardless of the area of subcutaneous fat the insulin is injected into. Any activity that speeds up blood flow, including exercise, can have such an effect. As a result, circulating insulin levels may increase during exercise but then be deficient later when insulin has been prematurely absorbed, especially with the use of intermediate or long-acting insulins. Some people use this increased absorption rate to their advantage to cause large decreases in blood sugar levels during exercise. If they start out with elevated blood sugars, they may take 0.5 to 3 units of Regular or Humalog insulin before beginning exercise to cause a rapid drop in blood sugars into a more normal range. The main danger of this practice is the possibility of taking more insulin than necessary and ending up hypoglycemic during the activity. Be cautious when using this technique. It is far better to underestimate the amount of insulin to take the first few times than to take too much and have a huge and rapid decrease in your blood sugars while you exercise.

SYMPTOMS OF HYPOGLYCEMIA

It is crucial for diabetic people to be aware of the variety of symptoms of hypoglycemia both at rest and during exercise. See table 3.2. A normal blood sugar range is from 70 milligrams per deciliter (mg/dl) (4 millimoles [mM]) to 110 mg/dl (6.1 mM). Technically, hypoglycemia can be defined as blood sugar below 70 mg/dl. However, the

Table 3.2 **Hypoglycemic Symptoms**

• Buzzing in ears	• Nausea
• Cold or clammy skin	• Nervousness
• Dizziness or lightheadedness	• Nightmares
• Double or blurred vision	• Poor physical coordination
• Elevated pulse rate	• Restlessness
• Fatigue	• Shakiness
• Hand tremors	• Slurred speech
• Headache	• Sweating
• Inability to do basic math	• Tingling of hands or tongue
• Insomnia	• Tiredness
• Irritability	• Visual spots
• Mental confusion	• Weakness

level of blood glucose that elicits symptoms of hypoglycemia can vary. If you have been in poorer metabolic control, sometimes you will get symptoms when blood sugars are above 70 mg/dl or while experiencing large drops in your blood sugar level without ever getting as low as 70 mg/dl. People with tighter control may not experience symptoms until reaching a much lower level (less than 55 mg/dl). Also, some people experience hypoglycemic unawareness, which means that they either do not have or recognize the usual symptoms. This condition appears to be more common in people with tight control. The usual symptoms of hypoglycemia include shakiness, hand trembling, tingling of hands or tongue, sweating, mental confusion, irritability, poor physical coordination (clumsiness), and visual changes; see table 3.2 for more symptoms. Activation of the sympathetic nervous system during exercise, which results in many of the hormonal changes, may result in some of the same symptoms as hypoglycemia, which activates a similar sympathetic nervous system response.

When performing certain types of exercise, people have reported having trouble distinguishing between the onset of symptoms of hypoglycemia and normal physical sensations associated with exercising, especially during exercise in cold weather. It may be difficult to distinguish between general fatigue resulting from exercise and fatigue resulting from the onset of hypoglycemia. Symptoms may also vary among people and different physical activities. One person with diabetes reports seeing a spot develop in one eye while

Zippora Karz

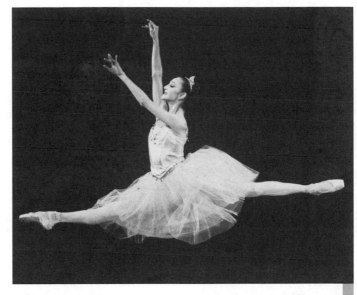

© Paul Kolnick/Choreography by George Balanchine

Zippora Karz was invited to the School of American Ballet (the official school of the New York City Ballet) at the age of 15 and to the New York City Ballet company at 18 in 1984. At 27, she became one of their 15 soloists. She was featured as the sugar plum fairy in *The Nutcracker* as well as soloist roles in Balanchine's *Apollo* and *Sleeping Beauty*.

At 21, Zippora was diagnosed with type 1 diabetes. Through trial and error, she learned to stay on top of her blood sugars when she danced. She said, "When dancing I had to be able to feel the tips of my toes. If my sugar wasn't right (too high or too low), I'd lose that vital connection." To prevent this, she tested her blood sugars almost hourly and adjusted her diet to keep her blood sugars on the high side of normal while dancing. During performances, she kept a blood glucose meter backstage to use before performing and during costume changes.

One time in her early years of performing with diabetes, she felt her blood sugars dropping severely right before a key performance. Her younger sister, also a member of the company then, noticed and helped her get some sugar quickly. Fortunately Zippora's blood sugars began to rise in time, but it was mid-performance before she no longer felt lightheaded. From that experience, she learned never to dose with any regular insulin before a performance. The NYC ballet management knew about her diabetes, but Zippora alone was responsible for maintaining her health and control despite a very physically active daily schedule. She had a 90-minute morning class, five-hour rehearsals for future ballets and the upcoming evening performance, and then the evening performance six days a week.

Although she chose to retire from professional ballet in 1999, she stays involved with dance by staging ballets for the George Balanchine Trust, while residing in Santa Fe, New Mexico. She still engages in her own dance workout regime daily. Her advice to young dancers with diabetes is this: "You can do it. You just have to go the distance with monitoring your blood sugars and controlling your diabetes."

running every time he becomes hypoglycemic, and another reports that he begins kicking the back of one heel with the other foot while running when his blood sugar level becomes too low. Some people just report a general sensation of fatigue, which can be difficult to distinguish from normal exercise fatigue. Symptoms may also change over time when fitness levels improve or worsen. It is crucial that you learn to recognize your own unique set of symptoms. Be aware that these symptoms can also vary with the type of exercise you do, the rate your low blood sugar occurs, and the environmental conditions (heat, cold, or altitude).

Chapter 4

Supplements and Eating for Exercise

As a physically active person, you are likely to be bombarded with claims about nutritional supplements that will enhance your athletic performance. With the fierce competition in sports, athletes look for any edge to improve their athletic abilities and will try almost any supplement or technique to get it—amino acid supplements, glycerol, sport drinks, creatine, carbohydrate loading, and ginseng, to name a few. In reality, very few of the advertised ergogenics for athletes are scientifically proven to enhance athletic prowess. Athletes with diabetes have special concerns about the effects of various supplements on diabetes as well as concerns about how to eat to effectively maintain blood sugar levels during exercise.

NUTRITIONAL SUPPLEMENTS

The list of advertised nutritional supplements that claim to enhance your athletic abilities is staggering. Most reports that appear to substantiate these claims are either studies done by the manufacturer of the product or anecdotes from people, often celebrities, who use the products. The problem for most athletes is determining which nutritional claims to believe. For more comprehensive coverage of all nutritional ergogenics refer to *The Ergogenics Edge: Pushing the Limits of Sports Performance* by Dr. Melvin Williams (Human Kinetics, 1998). This chapter discusses many, but not all, of the products listed in table 4.1 that receive the majority of hype and publicity and their actual effects on athletic performance and diabetes control.

Amino Acids

Have you ever heard that you have to take amino acid supplements to bulk up? Amino acids are the building blocks of proteins. Of the

Table 4.1 **Various Ergogenic Supplements Taken to Enhance Performance**

Nutritional	Pharmaceutical/physiological
Alcohol	Amphetamines
Antioxidants (vitamins C and E, beta-carotene, CoQ_{10}, and selenium)	Anabolic/androgenic steroids
	Androstenedione
Amino acids/branched-chain amino acids	Beta-blockers
Aspartates	Blood doping
B vitamins (niacin, riboflavin, thiamin, B_6, and B_{12})	Caffeine
	Cocaine
Caffeine	DHEA
Carnitine	Diuretics
Creatine	Ephedrine
Ginseng	rEPO
Glycerol	Human growth hormone
HMB	Insulin
Macronutrients (carbohydrates, fats, and protein supplements)	Marijuana
	Nicotine
Minerals (chromium, iron, magnesium, selenium, vanadium, and zinc)	Testosterone
Omega-3 fatty acids	
Phosphate salts	
Sodium bicarbonate	
Sport drinks	

20 different amino acids, nine are considered essential in the diet; you must ingest them through your diet or you will not have enough of them in your body. The remainder can be manufactured in the body and are considered nonessential in the diet (see table 4.2). You can buy practically every amino acid individually as a supplement, and many more are offered in combinations. Athletes have tried supplementing with practically all the amino acids to produce a per-formance-enhancing or strength-boosting effect.

The biggest myth about amino acid supplements, and protein in general, is that you have to load up on them to gain muscle mass. The protein requirement for strength-training athletes may be about twice as high as normal (1.6 to 1.8 grams of protein per kilogram of body weight daily instead of the usual recommended 0.8 grams), but most people in the United States already consume more than adequate amounts of protein in their normal diets. In order to gain one pound of muscle mass a week, a strength-training athlete would only need to eat an additional 14 grams of protein per day, which is easily attainable in less than two glasses of milk or two ounces of lean meat. The recommendation for endurance-training athletes is 1.2 to 1.6 grams of protein per kilogram of body weight per day (one kilogram equals 2.2 pounds). Athletes' requirements are likely higher than normal due to the large number of calories expended during prolonged endurance training.

Taking only specific supplemental amino acids may actually cause an imbalance of amino acids in your system by interfering with the absorption leading to an overabundance of some and a relative deficit of others. Excess calories ingested as amino acid supplements are simply converted to blood glucose or stored as excess fat. Furthermore, these supplements are expensive. An additional concern for people with diabetes is the load that excess protein consumption puts on the kidneys. Excess nitrogen in the form of urea must be excreted by the kidneys or sweat glands when excess protein is converted into other forms of energy in the body. Excretion of this excess urea is not usually a problem for healthy kidneys, but it can present an additional strain on kidneys with any damage from long-term diabetes. The bottom line is that taking amino acid

Table 4.2 **Amino Acids**

Essential amino acids	Nonessential amino acids
Histidine	Alanine
Isoleucine	Arginine
Leucine	Asparagine
Lysine	Aspartic acid
Methionine	Cysteine
Phenylalanine	Glutamic acid
Threonine	Glutamine
Tryptophan	Glycine
Valine	Proline
	Serine
	Tyrosine

Note: "Essential" amino acids are defined as those that cannot be manufactured in the body and must be included in the diet.

supplements is generally a waste of your money, and as a person with diabetes, you may actually be putting an additional strain on your kidneys. If you are determined to increase your intake of amino acids, simply increase your intake of healthy foods high in protein such as egg whites, nonfat milk, and lean meat.

Glycerol

Athletes have supplemented with glycerol (also called glycerin or glycerite), which is a simple compound that forms the backbone of triglycerides, your body's circulating and storage forms of fat. Glycerol has the capacity to attract water molecules to it, which leads to a superhydration effect. Dehydration can have a detrimental effect on performance in endurance activities because it can lead to early fatigue and more serious heat stress disorders. Glycerol is thought to exert ergogenic effects by increasing water retention and blood volume. As people with diabetes are more prone to dehydration (especially those with higher than normal blood sugars), supplementation with glycerol before exercising may help prevent this condition by loading the body with more water than normal. Of course, adequate fluid replacement (mainly water) during exercise is still vitally important even with glycerol use, especially if you exercise in a warm or hot environment. The recommended dose is 1 gram of glycerol per kilogram of body weight, diluted in other fluids, and consumed 1.5 to 2.5 hours before exercising. To date, there are no known side effects of glycerol supplementation at this dose.

Sport Drinks

Gatorade, PowerAde, All-Sport, Cytomax, GatorLode, Ultra Fuel—with so many sport drinks to choose from, how can you choose which one to use, if any? During physical activities, a fluid that is a 6 to 8 percent carbohydrate solution will empty from the stomach as rapidly as plain water and can effectively provide you with both water and carbohydrates. More concentrated solutions (above 10 percent carbohydrates) will empty less quickly from the stomach and should be ingested only before or following exercise rather than during an activity. Fruit juices are usually more concentrated than 10 percent and should be diluted for faster absorption if consumed during exercise. Drinks with high concentrations of fructose (fruit sugar) should generally be avoided during exercise, though, because they may cause gastrointestinal distress in the form of abdominal cramps or diarrhea. Table 4.3 lists various nutritional supplements, including sport drinks and glycerol, which may potentially benefit diabetic athletes.

Your need for sport drinks instead of water depends on the duration of an activity. For shorter events lasting an hour or less, you can effectively maintain hydration with water alone, although for athletes with diabetes, the extra carbohydrates in sport drinks or juice may be necessary to maintain blood sugar levels. Electrolyte replacement (sodium and potassium) is not necessary during these types of events because heavy sweating does not cause an immediate electrolyte imbalance. Sweat is actually more dilute than blood and contains less sodium and other electrolytes. For longer events, ingesting carbohydrate solutions has been shown to prolong endurance capabilities by providing an alternate carbohydrate energy source to maintain blood sugar levels in all athletes. Either a carbohydrate solution or water effectively maintains hydration. In very

Table 4.3 **Supplements of Potential Benefit to Diabetic Athletes**

Nutritional supplement	Potential beneficial effect
Antioxidants (vitamins C, E, beta-carotene, and selenium)	Reduction of oxidative damage to cell membranes induced by exercise and/or hyperglycemia
Carbohydrate, glucose intake	Intake of appropriate amounts of carbohydrate before, during, and after exercise to prevent hypoglycemia resulting from exercise
Chromium, vanadium, and zinc	Improvement in insulin sensitivity (especially in deficient type 2s)
Glycerol	Prevention of dehydration during exercise and when hyperglycemia is present
Sport drinks[a]	Prevention of hypoglycemia (if drink contains glucose or fructose) as well as dehydration and electrolyte imbalance during prolonged exercise, especially when done in the heat
Water, fluid replacement	Prevention of dehydration, especially due to hyperglycemia or exercise in the heat when perspiration is greater

[a]Sport drinks can also cause hyperglycemia if carbohydrate intake exceeds the necessary amount during exercise.

prolonged activities such as a full triathlon, some electrolyte replacement during the event may be beneficial as well to prevent dilution of the electrolytes in blood with large amounts of plain water, which causes a condition known as hyponatremia.

For the most effective hydration, it is good to take in fluids before starting an activity, during the activity, and following the activity. In general, the fluids should be cold and contain less than 10 percent carbohydrate for the best rates of gastric emptying. Research has also shown that drinking high volumes of any type of high-volume cold fluid may empty your stomach quickly. For example, 12 ounces of ice-cold water will empty from your stomach and get into your body for use more rapidly than half as much lukewarm water. You only need extra electrolytes if your activity is especially prolonged. It is also important to start drinking before you feel thirsty while exercising, because thirst is not triggered until you have already lost 1 to 2 percent of your body weight in the form of water.

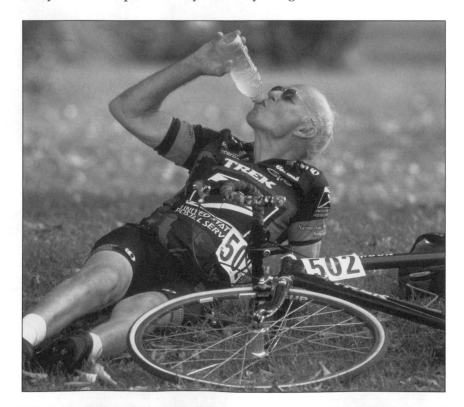

While water can keep you hydrated during exercise, sport drinks provide you with carbohydrates to maintain blood sugars as well.

Vitamins

Have you ever pictured yourself on the front of a box of Wheaties? And do you think that eating them every morning will make you a stronger, faster athlete? Many ordinary foods such as breakfast cereals, orange juice, and certain breads are now fortified with additional vitamins and minerals. Many athletes also take supplemental vitamins and minerals. Athletes supplement their diets with specific vitamins hoping to improve performance or enhance recovery. These vitamins include antioxidants and some of the B vitamins. B_{12} is the vitamin most commonly overused by athletes.

Antioxidants. The vitamins known collectively as antioxidants are vitamin C, vitamin E, and beta-carotene. Other supposed antioxidants are the mineral selenium and the compound CoQ_{10}. Antioxidant supplements are often sold as cocktails of all five of these combined. Exercise increases the production of oxygen-free radicals, which can damage cell membranes and other body structures. The human body produces some antioxidant enzymes that naturally squelch the majority of these free radicals. Antioxidant supplements are believed to help limit the cellular damage that may occur from oxidative free radicals produced during exercise. For people with diabetes, free radical production is increased by poor blood sugar control alone, making exercise an additional source of free radicals. While antioxidant supplementation has not been shown to directly increase sport performance, supplemental antioxidants may play a role in protecting muscles from cellular damage during strenuous training.

Antioxidant vitamins have different actions in the body. In addition to its antioxidant effect, vitamin C helps form the collagen that makes up connective tissues including ligaments and tendons. In addition, vitamin C aids in the absorption of iron from the gut and in the formation of the hormone epinephrine, which is released during exercise. Some people take large doses of vitamin C in an attempt to prevent the common cold and other viral infections. Vitamin C in a normal diet is found in citrus fruits, green leafy vegetables, broccoli, peppers, strawberries, and potatoes as well as in fortified products like Hi-C drinks.

Vitamin E helps to maintain the fluidity of red blood cell membranes as well as protect cell membranes throughout the body from oxidation. Dosages of up to 500 to 1,000 milligrams (mg) of vitamin C and 400 to 800 IU (International Units) of vitamin E do not appear to be harmful and may prevent damage from free radicals (see figure 4.1). A recent study of people with type 1 diabetes showed that high-dose vitamin E supplementation (1,800 IU a day) improves blood flow to the eye (retinal blood flow) and creatinine clearance (an indicator of normal kidney functioning) without significant changes in glycemic control. Vitamin E supplementation may, therefore, be especially beneficial for prevention of certain diabetic complications, although the exact recommended dosage has not yet been determined. Vitamin E is also recommended for athletes undergoing heavy training at high altitudes or in smoggy areas where oxidative stress may be greater. Vitamin E is a fat-soluble vitamin and is found naturally in vegetable oils, margarine, egg yolks, green leafy vegetables, wheat germ, and whole-grain products.

Supplements high in beta-carotene but low in vitamin A may also be beneficial as antioxidants. Both of these vitamins help maintain skin and mucous membranes, night vision, and proper bone development. Vitamin A is found in animal products such as liver, milk, and cheese, and beta-carotene is found in plants such as carrots and other yellow and orange vegetables. Vitamin A can be synthesized by the body as needed from beta-carotene, but it is best to avoid large doses of vitamin A; an overdose may be toxic.

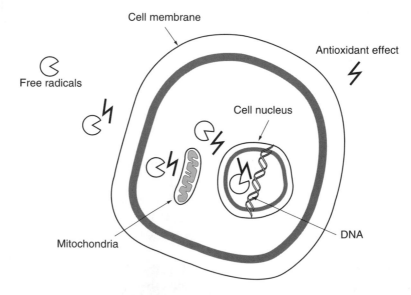

Figure 4.1 Antioxidant vitamins may help your body prevent some damage from free radical formation resulting from exercise and high blood sugars.

Vitamin B_{12}. Athletes use and abuse vitamin B_{12} with the belief that it enhances red blood cell production and, consequently, their oxygen-carrying capacity during endurance events. Some people have also used it in an attempt to increase their muscle mass. Although a deficiency of this vitamin could impair sport performance, no studies have shown that supplementing or even megadosing with it has an ergogenic effect on athletes who consume adequate amounts of vitamin B_{12} in their daily diets. It is found only in animal products (meat, dairy products, and eggs). Therefore, vegetarians, especially vegans (people who do not eat any meat or animal by-products), may benefit from B_{12} supplementation, but only if they do not consume enough vitamin B_{12} in their diets. However, vitamin B_{12} supplementation is generally not necessary or recommended.

Minerals

Minerals exert their effects on many energy pathways in the body due to their involvement with metabolism and enzymes involved in ATP production. Some mineral deficiencies would certainly have a negative effect on an athlete's exercise capacity. Diabetes itself can potentially cause certain mineral deficiencies. Among the minerals that diabetic athletes should consider supplementing are iron, calcium, magnesium, zinc, chromium, and vanadium.

Iron. Iron deficiency can affect the endurance performance of any athletic person. Iron forms part of the hemoglobin molecule that binds to and carries oxygen in the blood. Any reduction in hemoglobin reduces your oxygen-carrying capacity and oxygen delivery to working muscles and may limit your ability to do aerobic activities. Iron deficiency is a common problem, especially in endurance-trained athletes and women. Dietary iron is found in both animal and plant sources, but the iron in plants is absorbed more poorly through the gut than animal sources. If adequate iron is not present in the diet or absorption of iron is less than optimal, supplementation is recommended. Additional iron has not been found to enhance sport performance if body stores of iron are satisfactory.

Calcium. Although calcium intake does not directly affect sport performance, adequate amounts are crucial to the long-term health of your bones. Many older people experience osteoporosis (thinning of the bones), which greatly increases their risk for bone fractures. Both weight-bearing exercises and resistance training can stimulate the retention of more calcium in your bones. Calcium intake and absorption must be adequate, though, to maintain its content in bones. Sources of dietary calcium are all dairy products, egg yolks, dried beans and peas, broccoli, cauliflower, and dark green leafy vege-tables. Supplementing with calcium as well as foods rich in vitamin D to increase calcium absorption is recommended for any person with less than the recommended dietary intake. People with diabetes need to be especially diligent about taking in adequate amounts of calcium, because diabetes itself is known to cause a greater loss of bone mineral content.

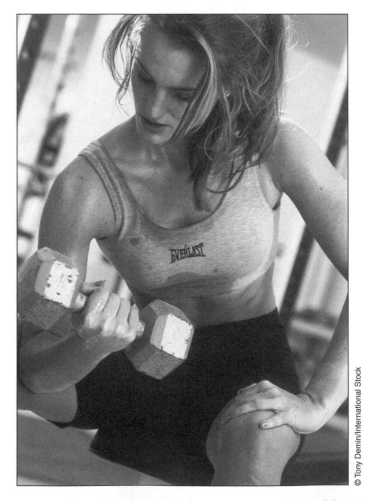

© Tony Demir/International Stock

Resistance training can help you prevent osteoporosis by stimulating calcium retention in your bones.

Magnesium. Several reports have recommended magnesium supple-mentation for people engaging in prolonged, intensive, regular physical training. However, the recommended increases still fall within the daily recommended intake levels. In the body, magne-sium is a component of more than 300 enzymes in skeletal muscle and bones. In muscle, it affects ATP utilization during contractions, oxygen metabolism, and glucose utilization. While a higher intake has not been found to improve sport performance, appropriate lev-els of magnesium may prevent muscle cramping and general muscle weakness. People with diabetes are more likely to be deficient in magnesium, so a proper dietary intake is recommended. Magne-sium is found in a variety of foods including nuts, seafood, green leafy vegetables, dairy, and whole-grain products.

Zinc. Zinc is a mineral that is involved in many body processes in-cluding wound healing, growth, protein synthesis, and immune functions. It is also a component of many enzymes involved in en-ergy metabolism including the lactic acid system and glucose me-tabolism. Low-calorie diets or excessive sweating may contribute to an excessive loss of zinc in people without diabetes. People with diabetes may be prone to deficiencies in this mineral due to impaired zinc absorption from the gut and excessive urinary losses of this mineral. One study of people with type 1 diabetes found that zinc supplementation of twice the recommended daily intake corrected zinc deficiency and improved the activity of a particular antioxi-dant enzyme. In other diabetic people, especially those with type 2 diabetes, zinc supplements reduced insulin resistance in muscle. Zinc supplementation has not been found to conclusively enhance mus-cular strength or athletic performance, though, and the intake of large doses of zinc may actually interfere with the normal intestinal absorption of other essential minerals such as iron and copper. Zinc should, therefore, not be taken in large doses, but people with dia-betes should consume adequate amounts of zinc through dietary intake of organ meats, poultry, seafood (especially oysters), dairy products, asparagus, spinach, and whole-grain products.

Chromium. Chromium is believed to enhance insulin sensitivity, lead-ing to improvements in blood sugar levels, storage of muscle and liver glycogen, and thus, performance in prolonged endurance ex-ercise. People with type 2 diabetes have taken large doses of chro-mium to improve their insulin action. Athletes have supplemented with chromium to increase lean body mass through the anabolic effects of insulin and to reduce body fat. No well-designed studies have shown increased chromium intake to have a significant effect on muscle and fat mass, muscular strength, or muscular endurance, however. Animal studies have shown that excessive amounts of this mineral may actually accumulate in cells and cause damage to DNA, but the long-term effects of supplementation in humans are not known. Chromium supplementation is only recommended for people who consume high-carbohydrate diets, exercise strenuously, or have an inadequate dietary intake of chromium. Dietary sources of chromium are organ meats, oysters, cheese, whole-grain products, asparagus, and beer. No more than the amount of chromium in a daily vitamin-mineral supplement is recommended (not to exceed 200 micrograms).

Vanadium. Vanadium (vanadyl sulfate) is a nonessential mineral that has also been used as an ergogenic aid by athletes. Some studies of humans have shown that supplementation with vanadyl salts can improve glucose metabolism in adults with type 2 diabetes because it may exert an insulin-like effect on glucose and protein metabolism. Vanadium is found in shellfish, grain products, parsley, mushrooms, and black pepper. Physicians may advise supplementation of vanadium to control blood glucose; however, it does not appear to have any effect on athletes' body composition or sport performances. You should not take excessive amounts of vanadium because it can be toxic to the liver and kidneys.

Caffeine

Caffeine is a stimulant found naturally in coffee, tea, cocoa, and chocolate. Caffeine directly stimulates the central nervous system and increases arousal. At the same time, it increases the levels of circulating epinephrine (adrenaline), which can mobilize free fatty acids (blood fats) and potentially provide an alternate fuel source for exercising muscles. It also stimulates the release of calcium in contracting muscles, which allows for greater force production and muscular strength. Research studies have found that caffeine increases performance in events that use each of the three energy systems: the ATP-CP system, the lactic acid system, and the aerobic system (see chapter 2 for a discussion of these systems). Legal doses of caffeine may improve running times in various distance events from one mile up to marathons. According to the International Olympic Committee, a legal amount is less than 800 mg depending on body weight. For comparison, a cup of coffee contains 100 to 150 mg, a cup of tea 50 mg, a can of cola 40 mg, a cup of cocoa 5 mg, a No Doz tablet 100 mg, and a Vivarin tablet 200 mg. You may be able to increase caffeine's effectiveness by abstaining from it for two to three days before a sport event; then on the day of the event, ingest caffeine before performing the activity. This causes you to be less habituated to its effects. The downside of caffeine is that it exerts a diuretic effect. When you ingest products that contain caffeine, you lose more water through urine than you would with products that do not contain caffeine. Hyperglycemia increases water loss as well. People with diabetes need to be especially cautious about maintaining proper hydration when ingesting caffeine, especially when exercising in a hot environment or when blood sugar levels are already elevated.

Creatine

Creatine is an amine present in animal products. It is formed in the liver and kidneys from other amino acids in your body. Normally, your daily dietary intake of creatine is 1 gram, and another gram is synthesized by your body as well. Creatine is present in all muscle cells both as free creatine and as creatine phosphate (CP), a main component of the phosphagen energy system (refer to chapter 2 for a discussion of this system). Many athletes have tried creatine monophosphate powder supplements to increase their performances in power sports. Oral supplementation has been found to increase the free creatine and CP stores in muscle as well as body weight mainly due to excess water retained in the muscle along with the extra creatine.

Many studies have found that creatine supplementation of 20 to 30 grams per day for five to seven days may exert an ergogenic effect on performance in explosive sports, primarily those that involve high-intensity, short-term, and repetitive exercise bouts with brief recovery periods. As a result, athletes may be able to train at a higher level, which could lead to an increase in muscle mass and gains in strength and power. The initial creatine-loading phase usually lasts for less than a week and is typically followed by a maintenance dose of 2 to 5 grams per day. Creatine supplementation has not been shown to enhance endurance performance and may be detrimental to distance running performance due to the resulting increase in body weight.

As of yet, there are no known long-term detrimental effects from creatine supplementation for nondiabetic people. However, excess creatine is excreted by the kidneys as creatinine, and in nondiabetic people, creatinine clearance levels have been shown to increase slightly during periods of creatine loading. No studies have examined the effects of creatine loading on people with diabetes. Diabetic athletes should be cautious in their use of this substance due to the additional stress placed on the kidneys caused by its excretion. Given the added health risks, if you choose to supplement, your intake should not exceed 20 grams per day for a period of five days (loading phase), with a subsequent intake of no more than 3 grams per day (maintenance phase). If you have kidney disease, as evidenced by an elevated creatinine clearance, microabuminuria, or overt proteinuria, supplementation with creatine is not advised.

Ginseng

Ginseng is derived from plants and is sold in different forms: Chinese or Korean, American, Japanese, and Russian/Siberian. Ginseng is believed to stimulate the hypothalamus, the brain's "control center" for several endocrine hormones that are released in your body. Ginseng is believed to accelerate recovery from exercise by enhancing the resynthesis of muscle glycogen and protein stores. It may also affect red blood cell hemoglobin levels and oxygen transport in the blood. Well-designed studies have not demonstrated these effects in athletes. However, one recent study showed that ingestion of American ginseng prior to a glucose load can significantly decrease an individual's blood glucose response to the ingested glucose. This study is the first to demonstrate any antidiabetic effect of ginseng. A concern is that an excessive intake may even worsen blood pressure problems in hypertensive diabetic individuals. Therefore, supplementation with ginseng is not recommended, especially for diabetic athletes with high blood pressure. Table 4.4 demonstrates supplements that are potentially harmful for diabetic athletes.

EATING FOR EXERCISE

No one likes to have to stop exercising because of low blood sugars. It can be especially inconvenient if you are out for a run or a long bike ride and are still a good distance from your destination and still

Table 4.4 **Supplements of Potential Harm to Diabetic Athletes**

Nutritional supplement	Potential harmful effect
Amino acid supplements	Amino acid imbalance in body, added stress on kidneys due to excess nitrogen excretion
Caffeine	Excessive water loss and dehydration especially during exercise in the heat
Carbohydrate loading[a]	Hyperglycemia before, during, and/or after exercise as well as reductions in insulin sensitivity; hypoglycemia if consumed before exercise and too much insulin is taken for carbohydrates
Creatine[b]	Added stress on the kidneys, especially if kidney disease is present, due to excess urinary excretion of creatinine
Fat loading	Slower carbohydrate absorption rates during exercise if consumed before or during activity, increased insulin resistance, ketone body production, and obesity in the long term
Protein supplements	Added stress on kidneys due to excess nitrogen excretion, especially when nephropathy is present

[a]Carbohydrate loading can also be beneficial to ensure proper replacement of muscle and liver glycogen levels before and after exercise. Adequate insulin must be available to prevent hyperglycemia and facilitate glucose uptake into muscle.

[b]Creatine will create the greatest kidney stress during the initial loading period (5-6 days). During the ensuing maintenance period of supplementation, added stress on the kidneys may be minimal if their functioning is normal.

have to get yourself there somehow. Preventing low blood sugar reactions during and following any activity is a high priority for all people with diabetes. You may have special concerns about how and what to eat to effectively maintain your blood sugar levels during and following exercise. In general, rapidly absorbed carbohydrates are most effective during exercise, but proteins and fats can be helpful after exercise as well. The following section includes some basic points to remember about effective use of the different energy sources.

Carbohydrate

Carbohydrate is the most important energy source for all forms of exercise. Muscle glycogen (the storage form of carbohydrates) is the primary source of energy for the lactic acid system as well as the

Bill Talbert

"He played to win in life."

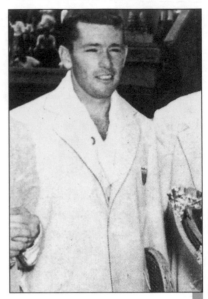

Bill Talbert was a successful professional tennis player who achieved 38 title wins in the 1940s and 1950s. While not a household name like Billy Jean King (who now also has diabetes) he certainly is an inspiration to anyone with diabetes. He was diagnosed with type 1 diabetes in 1928 at the age of 10, just seven years after the discovery of insulin. At that time, his doctor advised against participating in any activities that required lots of energy, so he took up marbles and became the best shooter in his neighborhood. At the age of 14, he received a tennis racket from his father and he started playing. Over the years of his professional tennis playing, he built his career on his ability to place a tennis ball exactly where he wanted it. He kept his hand in tennis long after he stopped playing at the top levels. He was a captain of the U.S. Davis Cup team from 1953 to 1957 and director of the U.S. Open Tennis Championships for another 15 years after that.

Playing competitive tennis with diabetes was a challenge in the days before blood glucose meters. Bill and his doctor came up with a "tennis diet" through trial and error that, most importantly, contained a bedtime snack to prevent overnight low blood sugars. With experience, he began to construct a game plan to work best with his diabetes. He had to depend on his accuracy and control of the tempo of the game to make sure that his body did not run out of energy reserves, especially when he faced opponents who played a power game. He said of his strategy, "When I walked onto the court for my opening round of play, I wasn't just starting a match, I was pursuing a health campaign."

After his tennis career, Bill donated much of his time to helping kids with diabetes through tennis camps and public speaking. He also excelled in his business ventures as executive vice president of the American Bank Note Company. Throughout his life, he maintained his active lifestyle by continuing to play tennis until the age of 68 and then continuing his active ways with walking daily and playing golf. When interviewed at the age of 72, he said, "My greatest accomplishment, I guess, is that I have survived as long as I have." When he finally passed away in 1998, he was in his 80th year and had lived an active, successful life despite having diabetes for 70 of those years.

main fuel for moderate to intense aerobic exercise. Ingested carbohydrates are broken down in your digestive tract and appear as blood glucose (your main blood sugar). The more intensely you exercise, the greater the rate you deplete glycogen stores in recruited muscle fibers. The liver also uses its glycogen stores to release glucose into the blood and maintain blood sugar levels during exercise. Depletion of muscle and liver glycogen stores during exercise will invariably lead to fatigue and force you to either stop exercising or slow down considerably.

In general, ingestion of carbohydrate is recommended for maintaining blood sugar levels during exercise due to its rapid metabolism and absorption compared to fat and protein. The type of carbohydrate needed depends on factors such as the duration of exercise, the intensity of your workout, and your blood sugar level before and during the exercise. Simple carbohydrate sources and those with a high glycemic index are absorbed more rapidly and have a more immediate effect on your blood sugar. The glycemic index of a carbohydrate refers to the rate of its absorption into your system and its effect on your blood glucose level. Some examples of recommended carbohydrates are juices, regular soda, sport drinks containing glucose or carbohydrate polymers, raisins, hard candies such as Lifesavers, bananas, and even bagels, bread, crackers, cornflakes, and potatoes. If you develop low blood sugar during exercise, one of these sources should be used for its treatment. In the general recommendations in part II of this book, the recommended carbohydrate intakes refer mainly to the more rapidly assimilated simple and high-glycemic-index carbohydrates as well. Other carbohydrate sources will not be as effective for immediate treatment of hypoglycemia due to their slower absorption rates. Although differences exist among people in their actual glycemic response, foods with a low glycemic index include high-fiber carbohydrates such as apples, cherries, dried beans and legumes (navy, kidney, chickpeas, lentils), dates, figs, peaches, plums, milk, and yogurt. Foods with a medium glycemic index include bananas, grapes, oatmeal, orange juice, pasta, rice, yams, corn, and baked beans. Carbohydrate-based foods with a high fat content have a slower absorption rate than carbohydrate-based food with a low fat content. Regular potato chips and doughnuts are examples of high-carbohydrate, high-fat foods; these carbohydrate sources would *not* be effective in the rapid treatment of hypoglycemia.

Carbohydrate supplementation may be an effective performance enhancer for athletes with or without diabetes. In general, research has demonstrated that carbohydrate supplementation during exercise is not necessary for events lasting an hour or less if muscle and liver glycogen stores are normal at the beginning of exercise. However, for maintenance of blood sugar levels during exercise, people with diabetes often need to take supplemental carbohydrate, even for exercise lasting less than an hour. All athletes who train frequently must have adequate amounts of carbohydrate on a daily basis to restore muscle and liver glycogen between training bouts. People

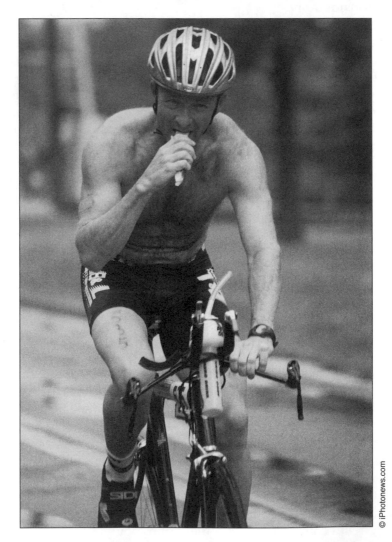

© iPhotonews.com

Supplementing with carbohydrates during exercise lasting an hour or more may improve an athlete's performance and delay the onset of fatigue.

with diabetes have to be even more careful about their blood sugar control following exercise in order for effective repletion to occur. For adequate glycogen storage, you must also have adequate insulin levels, especially more than an hour after exercise when glucose uptake into cells depends on insulin. Intake of higher-glycemic-index carbohydrates such as bagels or bananas immediately following exercise facilitates the initial muscle glycogen repletion, and in people with diabetes, early postexercise carbohydrate ingestion may also help lower the risk of hypoglycemia later on.

Carbohydrate supplementation during longer workouts or long sport events benefits all people. During marathons or triathlons, extra carbohydrate helps maintain athletes' blood sugar levels, enabling them to maintain a faster pace for a longer time. Extra carbohydrate intake has been shown to enhance playing ability for more intermittent, prolonged, high-intensity sports such as soccer, field hockey, and tennis. Therefore, you should take in adequate carbohydrate along with sufficient insulin before, during, and after prolonged, moderate, and high-intensity exercise to more effectively maintain and restore muscle and liver glycogen and blood glucose.

All athletes benefit from carbohydrate loading before long-distance events. Carbohydrate enables athletes to begin exercise with fully restored or even supercompensated muscle and liver glycogen stores. This loading technique usually consists of three to seven days of a high-carbohydrate diet combined with one to two days of rest or a reduction in exercise volume, which is known as tapering. Your daily diet should contain 8 to 10 grams of carbohydrate per kilogram of body weight, which is similar to endurance athletes's recommendations for carbohydrate intake. For carbohydrate loading to be effective for diabetic athletes, glucose uptake into muscle must be sufficient. You can ensure the proper replacement, and even supercompensation of muscle and liver glycogen, as long as you maintain a sufficient circulating level of insulin along with your carbohydrate intake to prevent hyperglycemia and facilitate glucose uptake. More high-fiber complex carbohydrates sources and those with a lower glycemic index will help prevent an excessive hyperglycemic response.

Fat

Both intramuscular and bloodborne lipids (fats) can be used as an energy source during exercise. Compared with carbohydrate, fat is a much more important energy source during low-intensity or prolonged activities such as walking the dog or taking an all-day hike. Exercise intensity largely determines the contribution of fat to ATP production. Plasma-free fatty acids (fats in blood) are first released from adipose (fat) tissue and then circulate to be taken up by muscle and used during low-level aerobic activities. During resting conditions, fatty acids can be stored as muscle triglycerides. For activities such as slow walking, circulating fat provides much of the energy for the activity. During moderate-intensity activities, more of the fat comes from intramuscular triglyceride stores, but only a small amount of fat is used along with a substantial amount of carbohydrate. Fat is not an optimal energy source for high-intensity aerobic or anaerobic exercise. During these activities, almost all energy is supplied by carbohydrate sources (muscle glycogen and blood glucose). During lesser-intensity or longer-duration exercise, fat can help spare blood glucose and muscle glycogen stores, especially when these energy sources become depleted, and fat provides much of the energy you use during recovery from exercise.

In general, a diet consisting of 30 percent or less of the total calories from fat is recommended for all people (see figure 4.2). A lower intake of saturated fat, which is fat that is solid at room temperature, trans fatty acids (such as those found in solid margarines), tropical oils (coconut, palm, and palm kernel oils), which are also high in saturated fat and cholesterol, may also help reduce the risk for heart disease. However, people with diabetes may use moderate fat in-

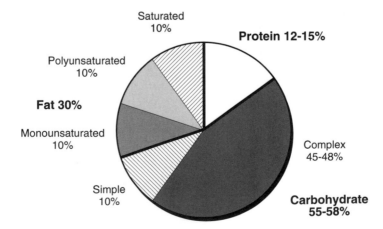

Figure 4.2 Exercise training and recovery require adequate intake of carbohydrate, protein, and fat in the approximate proportions recommended for all people.

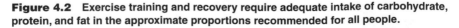

take after prolonged exercise as a means to prevent later-onset hypoglycemia. Many people may benefit from consuming a higher-fat bedtime snack following a day of prolonged or strenuous activity. Fat is metabolized much more slowly than carbohydrate and will provide an alternate energy source five to six hours following consumption. Fat loading (eating high-fat foods) for exercise may be detrimental to your performance. Fat consumed immediately before or during exercise will not be used for energy during that activity due to the longer time required for metabolism. High fat intake at these times is not recommended because it may also slow the absorption of ingested carbohydrates during exercise and contribute to obesity and insulin resistance long term.

Protein

Protein supplies up to 10 to 15 percent of all energy during a prolonged event such as a marathon, so it can also be used as an energy source, but it is not an important energy source for most short-duration exercise. Dietary protein is important, however, for muscle repair following strenuous exercise and for synthesis of hormones, enzymes, and other body tissues that are formed from amino acids (see the discussion of amino acids earlier in this chapter for the recommended protein amounts for various athletes). Protein synthesis during rest and recovery from exercise is vital to increases in strength, aerobic capacity, and size of muscles.

Some research has indicated that some protein intake along with carbohydrates immediately following depleting exercise may increase the resynthesis and storage of muscle and liver glycogen. For people with diabetes, some protein along with carbohydrate after an activity may prevent rapid drops in blood sugars. A bedtime snack containing some protein may also help prevent nocturnal hypoglycemia following a day of strenuous or prolonged activity. Protein intake immediately before exercise is not recommended, however, as the metabolism of protein occurs much more slowly than carbohydrate absorption.

Arguably the best nutritional ergogenic practice for individuals with diabetes is maintenance of the normal blood sugar levels during exercise. Abnormal blood sugars during an activity can impair your performance, typically by either causing you to fatigue (hypoglycemia) or by increasing your level of sluggishness (hyperglycemia). Carbohydrates need to be the most tightly regulated for exercise to prevent either of these conditions. Certain vitamins (B vitamins, antioxidants) and minerals (iron, calcium, selenium, chromium, vanadium) may affect your metabolism during exercise or may play a role in minimizing oxidative stress caused by exercise and diabetes. Caffeine ingestion may have an ergogenic effect during exercise, especially in individuals who are not habituated by its use. Creatine, while the latest nutritional ergogenic fad for athletes, should only be used with caution by people with diabetes due to the potential for extra stress on kidney function.

Chapter 5

Guidelines for Type 1 Diabetes

Many general exercise recommendations for athletes with type 1 diabetes now exist that can help them exercise more safely and effectively. This type of diabetes is generally caused by an autoimmune process that destroys the beta cells of the pancreas (where insulin is made). Individuals with type 1 diabetes must take insulin injections for the rest of their lives. Others with type 2 diabetes may start out making plenty of insulin and then later experience beta cell failure. At that point, they too would be dependent on insulin injections, although the etiology of their disease differs. The guidelines for type 1 diabetes apply to both of these groups of individuals as well as to any other users of insulin. In the earlier days of diabetes treatment, before blood glucose meters existed, physicians often advised their patients using insulin not to engage in physical exercise. Physical activity can increase your risk for hypoglycemia both during and after the activity, and it can even cause hyperglycemia, but you can exercise safely by following a few basic guidelines and safety precautions.

The American Diabetes Association (ADA) publishes clinical recommendations for exercise for people with type 1 diabetes. These guidelines, which have also been adopted by the American College of Sports Medicine (ACSM), focus on metabolic control before exercise, blood glucose monitoring before and after exercise, and food intake. Some physically active people with type 1 diabetes responded to a questionnaire about their exercise participation and normal regimen alterations (see appendix C). On this questionnaire, these people indicated their use of these current and past clinical exercise guidelines. Their possible responses to each guideline were as follows: 1 = I follow this guideline exactly; 2 = I follow this guideline most of the time; 3 = I follow this guideline sometimes; 4 = I follow this guideline very infrequently; and 5 = I follow this guideline almost never.

Table 5.1   **ADA and ACSM General Exercise Guidelines for Athletes With Type 1 Diabetes (and Other Insulin Users)**

Metabolic control before exercise

- Avoid exercising if fasting glucose levels are >250 mg/dl (14 mM) and ketosis is present, and use caution if glucose levels are >300 mg/dl (17 mM) and no ketosis is present.
- Ingest carbohydrates if glucose levels are <100 mg/dl (5.5 mM).

Blood glucose monitoring before and after exercise

- Identify when changes in insulin or food intake are necessary.
- Learn the glycemic response to different exercise conditions.

Food intake

- Consume carbohydrate as needed to avoid hypoglycemia.
- Keep carbohydrate-based foods readily available during and after exercise.

CURRENT GUIDELINES

Due to the possibility of worsening metabolic control during exercise (resulting in either hyperglycemia or hypoglycemia), the guidelines address the areas of metabolic control, blood glucose monitoring, and food intake for physical activity. See table 5.1 for current ADA and ACSM guidelines.

Metabolic Control Before Exercise

The two general guidelines concerning metabolic control before exercise and athletes' responses address conditions of hyperglycemia and potential hypoglycemia. The first guideline states that people should avoid exercising if fasting glucose levels are more than 250 mg/dl (14 mM) and ketosis is present and use caution if glucose levels are more than 300 mg/dl (17 mM) and no ketosis is present. (The guideline that athletes were questioned about was actually the previous version of this one, which stated that exercise should not occur for blood sugars above 300 mg/dl, irrespective of whether ketosis was present.) The responses to this guideline varied: about 40 percent of athletes said that they follow this guideline exactly or most of the time, and another 40 percent said that they follow this very infrequently or almost never. The 1999 version of this guideline was the least followed one of the current recommendations.

As justification for their noncompliance, some athletic people stated that they either have never experienced ketosis or just never check their urine for ketones, while others stated that their fasting blood sugar is never that high or that their blood sugars are only that high for a very short period of time. The majority of athletes who do not follow this guideline either find that exercise itself always reduces their blood sugars or that exercise can be combined with a small dose of short-acting insulin. For the people who simply exercise anyway, many commented that they know the reason for their blood sugar increase is that they have just eaten a meal and that exercise always helps to normalize their blood sugars, regardless of the level, as long as they have taken their usual insulin.

Many other athletes commented about their use of supplemental insulin to reduce their blood sugar levels during exercise. A common practice is to administer 1 to 2 units of rapid-acting insulin (preferably Humalog) before exercising, wait 10 to 15 minutes, and then begin normal exercise. For most people, the combination of insulin and exercise brings their blood sugars down to normal by the end of the activity. The main danger of this practice is the possibility of overestimating your insulin needs, which results in hypoglycemia during the activity. The usual decrease in blood glucose elicited by exercise combined with a recent injection of short-acting insulin can cause an abrupt onset of hypoglycemia. Be cautious if you use this technique; it is far better to underestimate a supplemental insulin dosage than to experience a precipitous drop in your blood sugars and be forced to contend with rapid-onset hypoglycemia while you exercise.

A minority of athletes commented that they actually follow this guideline and avoid exercising. However, when ketones are a result of illness or infection, most athletes do not exercise until they recover from illness or infection and their blood sugars are under better control. When ketosis is present due to severe insulin deficiency, exercise can cause an increase in blood sugar levels and lead to the development of diabetic ketoacidosis, a potentially serious and life-threatening condition that usually requires hospitalization.

The second guideline concerning metabolic control states the following: Ingest added carbohydrates if glucose levels are less than 100 mg/dl (5.5 mM). The majority of people (78 percent) reported that they follow this guideline exactly or most of the time. Their comments indicated that while many people follow this guideline exactly many others modify it depending on other factors. Some of these factors include how much exercise time remains, how much insulin they took and how long before exercising they injected it, the type of exercise they engage in, how hard they work out, the expected duration of the activity, and even the environmental conditions (hot weather may cause blood sugars to fall lower than usual). For intense exercise such as weight training, many people commented that they did not need extra carbohydrates, but they follow this guideline for more prolonged, less intense activities. The time of day of the activity also makes a big difference to many people. For example, morning exercise requires less adjustment than other times of day. Depending on the activity, some people try to eat enough to increase their blood sugars to a certain level (e.g., 150 to 180 mg/dl) before the activity to prevent hypoglycemia during exercise. For others, the personal cutoff level may be 75 mg/dl instead of 100 to supplement with carbohydrate. Other athletes, especially insulin pump users who can modify their basal insulin rates, often choose to reduce their insulin instead of eating extra carbohydrates.

Blood Glucose Monitoring

Two other guidelines address the issues around blood glucose monitoring practices. The first guideline recommends the following: Identify when changes in insulin or food intake are necessary. The vast majority of people (82 percent) reported that they follow this guideline exactly or most of the time. Many people indicated that they feel glucose monitoring is essential in establishing a pattern and making changes. Others commented on the insulin or food alterations they have learned to make mostly through trial and error. One athlete commented, "If possible, I check two hours before, then one hour before, then just before (exercise) so I know if I'm going up or down. Then I test immediately when I finish and eat carbohydrate if needed." Most athletes will check their blood sugars at least before and after exercise, and many more even test during an activity. In general, people find that they need more testing for new and unusual exercise than for established routines. Athletes make insulin and food changes depending on their insulin regimens and other factors such as intensity and type of exercise.

The second guideline states that diabetic exercisers should learn the glycemic response to different exercise conditions. Seventy-three percent of athletic people reported that they follow this guideline exactly or most of the time. Many differentiated their responses by the type of exercise, whereas others voiced their frustrations with attempting to establish definite patterns. In general, athletes indicated that anaerobic and shorter-duration aerobic exercise require fewer modifications than prolonged aerobic activities. As for establishing a definite pattern, one triathlete commented, "When learning how my body responds, I check my blood glucose every hour, all waking hours, to find any changes in blood glucose from which I can learn by tracking the activity and its effect." Athletes' frustrations are that there are too many variables for perfect prediction, although general trends are predictable for most activities. Establishing a trend usually involves a lot of trial and error. Active people generally agree that the best way to deal with the multitude of variables that affect your blood sugar is to learn your own responses to all of them by checking blood sugar levels before, during, and after exercise. Hopefully, a somewhat predictable pattern will emerge to help you anticipate your responses to future bouts of similar exercise.

Food Intake

The last two guidelines address carbohydrate intake related to exercise. In response to the guideline that states that people should consume carbohydrate as needed to avoid hypoglycemia, over 90 percent of people reported that they follow this guideline exactly or most of the time. Athletes indicated which types and amounts of carbohydrates they consume for various types of exercise as well as modifications they make in carbohydrate intake or insulin dosages. People consume rapidly absorbed carbohydrates to prevent and treat hypoglycemia (see chapter 4) including regular soda, sport drinks, juice, hard candy, glucose tablets, dried fruits, skim milk, bread, and carbohydrate bars. The amount of carbohydrates they eat depends on timing and doses of insulin, type of activity, and starting blood sugar levels. Other exercisers prefer to adjust their insulin dose instead of consuming extra food. Most of the people who gave this response use an insulin pump; pump users can readily lower or discontinue basal insulin intake during an activity.

The second recommendation is as follows: Carbohydrate-based foods should be readily available during and after exercise. Almost 93 percent follow this guideline exactly or most of the time. Most people commented that they carry extra carbohydrates with them during exercise. Very few people exercise without having these available at all times.

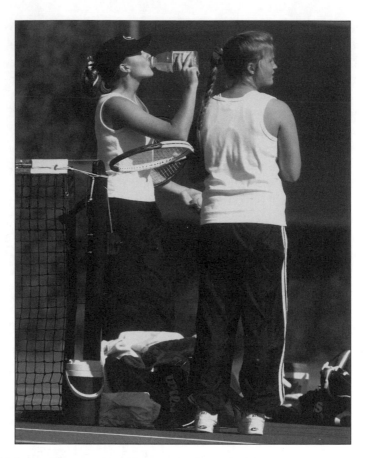

Sport drinks contain enough rapidly-absorbed carbohydrates that you can use them to prevent and treat low blood sugars.

PREVIOUS GUIDELINES

Some of the previously published guidelines also addressed carbohydrate and insulin changes for prolonged and strenuous exercise as well as injection sites and time of day exercise is done. In general, athletes follow these older guidelines much less stringently than the current guidelines, probably due to improvements in insulin regimen choices, the ability to monitor blood sugars, and other advances in diabetes care. However, the older (more outdated) recommendations were also more specific about amounts of carbohydrate to ingest and insulin changes to make than the current exercise recommendations are.

Carbohydrate Intake

Athletic diabetics were previously advised to ingest 15 to 30 grams of carbohydrate for every 30 minutes of intense exercise. The majority of athletes follow this recommendation sometimes (24 percent), very infrequently (20 percent), or almost never (23 percent), leaving only a third to follow it exactly or most of the time. Some athletes think this amount is too much, some think it is too little, some think it is just right, and the rest think it depends on a number of variables. Among these variables are the type and intensity of exercise, exercise duration, circulating insulin levels, the results of blood glucose monitoring, and the insulin regimen. Their most common response about how much carbohydrate to ingest was, "It depends." Most athletes rely on the results of blood sugar monitoring to make modifications to carbohydrate intake. Other people do not follow this guideline because they exercise consistently and make corrections by modifying their insulin doses. As one athlete remarked, "All people are different; therefore, the amount of [carbohydrate] grams will vary as well as the frequency of ingestion. The key is to have enough insulin on board so your glucose level does not increase with exercise without ingestion and to learn the amount of carbohydrates to ingest."

A second guideline recommended that people consume a snack of carbohydrate soon after exercising. Most people (37 percent) follow this guideline sometimes or most of the time (27 percent). Many reported that they eat a meal soon after exercise, so it is not really a snack but a regularly scheduled meal. The majority of comments indicated that snacking after exercise depends on blood sugar levels. The rest of the comments indicated that snacking depends on other factors such as preexercise insulin doses and circulating insulin levels at the end of exercise.

Insulin Regimen Adjustments

Four previous guidelines for adjusting insulin doses were categorized by insulin regimen. The first guideline addressing intermediate-acting insulin referred mainly to doses of NPH or Lente but applied to Ultralente as well. It stated that athletes should decrease their doses of intermediate-acting insulin by 30 to 35 percent on the day of exercise. Almost two-thirds of people reported following this guideline sometimes or most of the time. The majority of reported dose reductions frequently varied from the recommended 30 to 35 percent decrease, however. Many people still take close to their usual dosage of NPH or Lente for normal daily activities and only make larger adjustments for unusual activities such as all-day hiking or cross-country skiing. Other athletes indicated that they may reduce their bedtime doses following the activity but they don't adjust their morning doses prior to exercising. Others only take intermediate-acting insulins at bedtime and do not make changes to those doses. Yet other athletes choose to compensate for activities with increased carbohydrate intake alone.

The second recommendation addressed insulin omission. It recommended that doses of intermediate-(NPH or Lente) and short-acting insulins (Regular insulin or Humalog) be omitted if they normally precede exercise. Almost half (46 percent) of all people stated that they follow this guideline almost never, 14 percent stated that they follow it very infrequently, and another 14 percent sometimes follow it. The majority of people stated that they do not omit the dose; they only reduce it. The most common comment was that complete omission of these doses before exercise results in elevated blood sugars, but reductions both preceding and following exercise often work well in preventing low blood sugars.

The third guideline addressing multiple doses of short-acting insulin applied mainly to Ultralente, NPH, or Lente users who dose with short-acting insulins for all meals and snacks during the day. Users of these regimens were advised to reduce the short-acting insulin dose before exercise by 30 percent and supplement with carbohydrate intake. Almost one-third (29 percent) reported following this guideline almost never, while 20 percent follow it sometimes, and 22 percent follow it most of the time. However, the majority of people did indicate that they make reductions in their insulin; they just vary from the recommended 30 percent reduction, depending on variables such as the intensity and duration of exercise, starting blood sugar levels, levels of circulating insulin during the activity, and carbohydrate intake. One athlete commented, "When I do high-intensity exercise, my insulin sensitivity doubles if I've just had a shot. I try to keep shots away from exercise."

The final guideline on continuous subcutaneous insulin infusion applied to insulin pump users. They were advised to eliminate their mealtime bolus or insulin increment that precedes or follows exercise. Over half of insulin pump users stated that they follow this guideline almost never or very infrequently; they simply reduce the

Steve Prosterman

"He has opened up the underwater world to many individuals with diabetes."

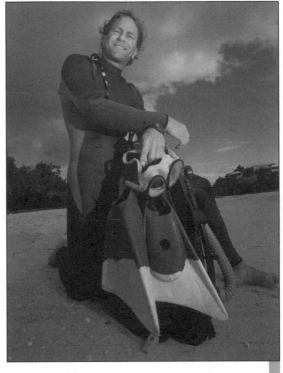

© Steve Simonsen

Steve Prosterman is not a famous athlete or a household name; he is a recreational athlete who exercises daily by swimming, scuba diving, windsurfing, sea kayaking, sailing, playing basketball, weight training, or cycling. He is also a scuba-diving instructor in the marine biology department at the University of the Virgin Islands in St. Thomas. For the past 10 years, he has also been organizing and running a one-week activity camp every summer for adults with diabetes (Camp DAVI). In doing so, he has enabled people with diabetes to safely explore the underwater world of the Caribbean through scuba diving.

Diagnosed with type 1 diabetes at the age of nine, Steve has never let it keep him from doing the things he enjoys. Fresh out of college he traveled to the U.S. Virgin Islands in 1979 at the age of 22, looking for adventure. While teaching school there, he became interested in scuba diving from a friend who was an underwater photographer. He became PADI certified in scuba diving and instructing (before most diabetic people were banned or discouraged from diving).

Steve started DAVI (Diabetes Association of the Virgin Islands), an educational support organization not affiliated with the ADA, and later Camp DAVI, which he still coordinates single handedly. He has come up with many safety techniques for diabetic divers to use to prevent hypoglycemia while scuba diving. He has also worked with DAN (the Divers Alert Network) to assist them in conducting studies to demonstrate the safety of scuba diving for people with diabetes. He personally engages in all of his water activities with a tube of InstaGlucose tucked in his swimming suit.

Steve is full of energy. He never lets diabetes get in the way of his enjoyment of life. Despite his many activities, he often recreates by swimming with the dolphins in the warm waters of the Caribbean Sea, and he finds time to play with his three-year-old daughter who is into sea kayaking with her dad. He is also known around St. Thomas for his less serious hobbies: juggling fire torches and knives while eating an apple and riding a six-foot unicycle around town.

dose preceding or following exercise but almost never omit it completely. Other pump users alternately or additionally lower or eliminate basal insulin rates during the exercise. One athlete commented, "I do not eliminate my mealtime bolus. I might reduce it depending on blood sugar reading and exercise factors such as duration and heat." Another person's guideline is "High intensity, lower boluses. Low intensity, lower boluses and lower basal." Other athletes indicated that they may eliminate a usual snack bolus during the activity.

Injection Sites and Timing of Exercise

Another previous recommendation addressed the choice of insulin injection sites before physical activity. The guideline advised people to avoid exercising for one hour those muscles that short-acting insulin was injected into. Over half of the athletes (55 percent) reported that they follow this recommendation almost never. Only 17 percent reported that they follow it exactly. Other people brought up a good point about this guideline: Insulin is not usually injected into a muscle; it's injected into subcutaneous fat (the fatty layer below the surface of the skin)! However, if insulin is to be injected into a limb with very little fat, it may be best to avoid that area prior to exercising. For those athletes who do not follow it, many felt it does not apply to them because they only use their abdomen for administration of all types of insulin. Most athletes said that they cannot tell a difference with different injection sites, while only a limited number of people stated that they notice a difference and are very careful where the insulin is injected before exercise. Research has actually shown that exercise can increase insulin absorption rates from any subcutaneous depot, so your choice of insulin injection site is probably not going to affect the potential increase in circulating insulin levels that result from exercising.

A final previous recommendation was to avoid exercising in the late evening, presumably to reduce the risk of nocturnal hypoglycemia (low blood sugars during the night). One-third of the people reported following this guideline almost never, with the rest almost evenly split among all the other possible responses. For many of those who follow this guideline, they stated it was because of their personal preference of when to exercise, not for diabetes-related reasons. The most common reason for not adhering to this guideline was the logistics of finding time to exercise earlier in the day. As one exerciser commented, "I fit exercise in whenever I can. Sometimes it ends up being late, but I'd never consider not exercising in the later evening because I have diabetes." Many also commented on precautions or concerns that they have for evening exercise. These precautions include eating an extra bedtime snack or lowering their insulin doses overnight.

ADA/ACSM STATEMENT ON GUIDELINES

While athletic people with type 1 diabetes obviously have already recognized the inappropriateness of some of these previous guidelines, the *Clinical Practice Recommendations* also include the following statements, which recognize the ineffectiveness of some of these previous recommendations.

"The ability to adjust the therapeutic regimen (insulin and medical nutrition therapy) to allow safe participation and high performance has recently been recognized as an important management strategy in these individuals (people with type 1 diabetes). In particular, the important role played by the patient in collecting self-monitored blood glucose data of the response to exercise and then using these data to improve performance and enhance safety is now fully accepted." In addition, they state, "The rigid recommendation to use carbohydrate supplementation, calculated from the planned intensity and duration of exercise, without regard to glycemic level at the start of exercise, the previously measured metabolic response to exercise, and the patient's insulin therapy, is no longer appropriate. Such an approach not infrequently neutralizes the beneficial effects of exercise in patients with type 1 diabetes."

EXERCISE PRECAUTIONS

People with diabetes who are in good metabolic control and do not have serious diabetic complications can engage in any type of exercise, whether a professional sport or a recreational physical activity. However, some valid concerns exist that are more relevant to people with diabetes, such as the potential for hypoglycemia during and following the activity, hyperglycemia, and dehydration. Actual problems may arise when a person has diabetes-related complications. The following are some of the more salient concerns and recommended precautionary measures.

Prevention of Hypoglycemia or Hyperglycemia Following Exercise

Hypoglycemia can occur during or after exercise and is preventable with appropriate changes in insulin and food intake. Consuming carbohydrates after exercise allows for more efficient repletion of muscle glycogen stores and may actually help prevent postexercise late-onset hypoglycemia, which can occur up to 24 hours following exercise. To optimize repletion of glycogen following exhaustive, depleting exercise (either repeated bouts of high-intensity or long-duration exercise), it is best to consume carbohydrates within 30 minutes after exercise. During this time, uptake of glucose into muscle to reform glycogen can be accomplished with a minimal amount of insulin in the body as insulin sensitivity is heightened. Furthermore, with more effective glycogen repletion early on, there is less of a risk for late-onset hypoglycemia. Monitor blood glucose levels at one-hour intervals after exercise to make adjustments in insulin or food to prevent hypoglycemia or hyperglycemia. A low-carbohydrate intake after exercise or carbohydrate intake without sufficient insulin (although a lower insulin dose is usually necessary) may compromise or delay the normal course of glycogen repletion after exhaustive exercise.

Prevention of Dehydration

People with diabetes may be more prone to dehydration than people without diabetes, especially when higher blood sugar levels cause more water loss in urine (polyuria) or in people with autonomic neuropathy. Autonomic neuropathy is a chronic complication of diabetes affecting the autonomic nervous system that may cause an abnormal cardiac function (heart rate changes), dizziness upon standing, or impaired movement of food through the digestive system. Dehydration may not be immediately evident because thirst centers are not activated until a 1 percent or more loss of body water has occurred. You should be adequately hydrated before exercise, and you should drink fluids early and frequently to compensate for sweat losses during exercise. Cool, plain water is the recommended beverage for fluid replacement before, during, and after short-term moderate exercise (up to 60 minutes). Diabetic exercisers may need water and extra carbohydrates for exercise lasting longer than 60 to 90 minutes. Diluted fruit juices and sport drinks are good sources of

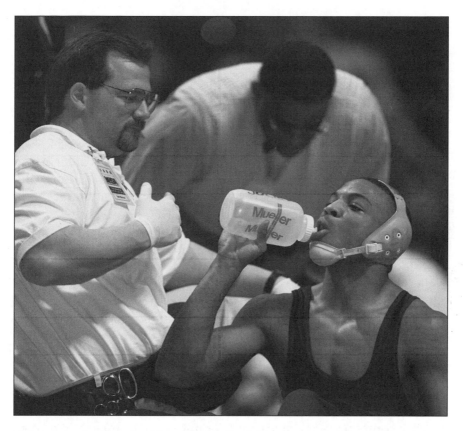

Plain, cool water is the best for replacing the fluids you lose during shorter activities.

both water and carbohydrates. You should continue to drink extra fluids following an activity as it takes up to a day to fully restore fluids lost through sweat and ventilation.

Exercise With Complications

For a comprehensive coverage of potential diabetes-related complications, refer to a publication by the American Diabetes Association, *The Health Professional's Guide to Diabetes and Exercise* (1995). Complications can be either microvascular or macrovascular in origin. Microvascular complications include neuropathies (peripheral and autonomic), retinopathy, and nephropathy. Macrovascular concerns may involve heart or peripheral vascular disease and hypertension.

Peripheral neuropathy. For those people with some peripheral loss of sensation, risk of foot damage is greater as nerve damage can blunt signals of pain or discomfort from high impact on the feet or friction or pressure from footwear. The ADA recommends the use of silica gel or air midsoles in shoes as well as polyester or blend (cotton-polyester) socks to prevent blisters and keep the feet dry to minimize trauma resulting from exercise. Proper footwear is also essential for prevention of problems. Non-weight-bearing exercises are recommended to improve tone, balance, and awareness of the lower extremities. Recommended exercises include swimming, pool walking, water aerobics, stationary bicycling, rowing, arm ergometer work, upper-body exercises, t'ai chi, and other non-weight-bearing activities. Range of motion exercises can also help prevent contracture of the lower limbs. Contraindicated exercises may include weight-bearing activities such as prolonged walking, jogging, treadmill exercise, and step exercises. People with neuropathic changes must also monitor their feet closely both before and after exercise for blisters and other potential damage. Exercise cannot reverse peripheral neuropathy, but it can slow its progression and prevent further loss of fitness resulting from inactivity.

Autonomic neuropathy. People with autonomic system nerve damage are at high risk for developing complications during exercise, including silent myocardial infarction and sudden death when the heart becomes unresponsive to autonomic nerve impulses. Hypotension (low blood pressure) can occur more easily with rapid changes in body position in these people. With autonomic neuropathy, people can also have difficulty maintaining normal body temperatures and levels of hydration and should avoid exercising in hot or cold environments. With orthostatic hypotension, dizziness or fainting with changes in body position are much more possible and rapid changes are best avoided. With gastroparesis, any foods taken to treat or prevent hypoglycemia during exercise may have a delayed or uneven absorption, resulting in first low and later high blood sugar levels during exercise and recovery. Because this metabolic response to exercise can vary widely, blood sugar monitoring is essential for effective and safe exercise for these people. Autonomic neuropathy may also increase the likelihood of insulin-induced hypotension, which tends to be worse in the morning. A conservative approach to exercise is best for these people. Exercise intensity is best monitored using the Rating of Perceived Exertion (RPE) scale as autonomic neuropathy can blunt maximal and submaximal heart rates.

Proliferative retinopathy. This is the process of formation of weak, abnormal blood vessels in the back of the eye (retina) that can break, tear, or bleed into the vitreous fluid, filling the eye. In general, exercise has not been shown to accelerate the proliferative process. However, certain precautions may be appropriate, depending on the level of retinopathy. With moderate proliferation, activities that dramatically increase blood pressure should be avoided. These include heavy weightlifting, powerlifting, or heavy Valsalva maneuvers. For more severe retinopathy or active hemorrhaging, it is best to avoid activities that cause a large increase in systolic blood pressure or involve pounding and jarring, including boxing, heavy competitive sports such as basketball or football, weightlifting, jogging, high-impact aerobics, racket sports, and strenuous trumpet playing. These activities increase the risk of retinal tears, retinal detachment, and vitreous hemorrhage. Among the recommended activities are exercises such as swimming, walking, low-impact aerobics, stationary cycling, and other endurance exercises done at a low to moderate level.

Nephropathy. In the early stages of kidney disease, there is some evidence that exercise can increase rates of albumin excretion in the urine. However, there is no evidence that regular endurance activity speeds progression of the disease. Exercise may also increase albumin excretion in diabetic individuals without kidney disease (through exercise-induced proteinuria), so for accurate results on your kidney function, it is best not to exercise during a 24-hour urine collection done to assess the microalbumin and protein content in your urine. Severe or excessive exercise is usually not recommended for people with overt nephropathy, usually because their exercise capacity is limited. Light to moderate exercise is fine for these people, though. Patients on dialysis can often exercise on a stationary cycle during the treatments with no ill effects. Exercise for these people is only contraindicated if hematocrit, calcium, or phosphorus blood levels are unstable due to the need for dialysis. Diabetics who have undergone renal transplantation may safely exercise six to eight weeks after the transplant when they are stable and free of rejection.

Heart disease. Exercise decreases cardiac risk, but people with diabetes are still at higher risk than the general population for cardiovascular complications. Exercise has positive effects on insulin sensitivity and lipid metabolism. It can improve the lipoprotein profile, reduce blood pressure, and improve the fitness of the cardiovascular system as a whole. Exercise-induced ischemia (decreased blood flow to the heart) may be asymptomatic in people with diabetes when any degree of autonomic neuropathy is present. The ADA recommends a graded exercise test before participation in moderate- to high-intensity exercise for people at higher risk, including people with diabetes over the age of 35, type 1 diabetes longer than 15 years, type 2 diabetes longer than 10 years, additional risk factors for cardiovascular disease, microvascular disease (retinopathy or nephropathy including microalbuminaria), peripheral vascular disease, or autonomic neuropathy. Those with known cardiovascular problems should exercise in a medically supervised environment where monitoring is available. For people with these risk factors, an exercise program should start with low-intensity aerobic exercise and progress slowly. An exercise stress test should be performed periodically to test for the ischemic threshold so that exercise can be done at a lower level to minimize risks for cardiovascular events or arrhythmias. Heavy weight training is contraindicated due to the excessive strain it places on the heart and vasculature.

Hypertension. Exercise training helps lower chronic high blood pressure. Moderate-intensity aerobic exercise is generally recommended for those people with elevations in blood pressure. Weight training can also be done as long as the focus is on low-weight, high-repetition training, which would cause less dramatic increases in blood pressure than heavy weightlifting. High-intensity (near maximal effort), isometric exercises, and the Valsalva maneuver (breath-holding) should be avoided due to their ability to cause extreme increases in systolic and diastolic blood pressures.

Despite the potential risks associated with exercise, the benefits to people with diabetes generally far outweigh the risks.

So no matter what, find a way to exercise as much as you are capable of doing! Take precautions where necessary, especially if you have any complications. For example, avoid doing heavy weight training if you have active retinal hemorrhages. You can safely participate in less strenuous forms of exercise. You can learn to manage your blood sugars effectively during any type of physical activity. Remember, the best way to deal with the multitude of variables that affect blood sugar and your response to exercise is to learn your own responses to all of them by checking blood sugar levels before, during, and after exercise.

Chapter 6

Guidelines for Type 2 Diabetes

Many reports indicate that the increasing incidence of type 2 diabetes is associated with a decreasing level of physical activity and an increasing prevalence of obesity. Type 2 diabetes is essentially an insulin-resistant condition. Many times blood sugars can be controlled with diet and exercise alone, at least initially. Oral hypoglycemic agents and other diabetic medications are used when blood sugars begin to no longer be controlled with this regimen. Weight loss often times improves blood sugar control as well. Exercise can be a vital component in the prevention and management of type 2 diabetes when used in conjunction with diet, oral medication, and insulin therapies. If insulin is used for type 2 diabetes treatment, the guidelines given for type 1 apply as well (refer to chapter 5). Abnormalities in insulin sensitivity (ineffective insulin action in muscle and fat tissues) can be lessened with regular physical activity. The potential benefits of exercise for people with type 2 diabetes are, therefore, enormous. To make exercise safe and effective for all, some general guidelines apply as well as some safety precautions.

EXERCISE GUIDELINES

Exercise guidelines for people with type 2 diabetes differ somewhat from those for active people with type 1 simply due to the differences in the origin of the diabetes. Type 1 athletes have to take insulin injections, whereas only a minority of type 2 athletes use insulin. The majority of type 2 athletes use a combination of diet, exercise, and oral hypoglycemic agents to control their blood sugars and lessen their state of insulin resistance. The age of onset is often very different as well. Because they are usually older, athletes with type 2 diabetes may need a preexercise evaluation by their physicians to ensure that exercise will not worsen any other existing health problems. They, like type 1 athletes, will benefit from frequent blood glucose monitoring to determine the effects of exercise, although hypoglycemia is not as great of a risk and the chances of developing ketosis from a relative insulin deficiency are minimal.

Preexercise Medical Evaluation

Most people with type 2 diabetes wishing to engage in moderate to vigorous exercise should first undergo a detailed medical evaluation that includes screening for the presence of macrovascular or microvascular complications that could be worsened by exercise. These complications include heart or peripheral vascular disease and nerve, eye, or kidney changes. For example, significant peripheral neuropathy (loss of sensation in the feet) would necessitate limiting weight-bearing exercise and focusing more on non-weight-bearing activities. The presence of autonomic neuropathy may limit a person's exercise capacity and increase the risk for cardiovascular events during exercise. Orthostatic hypotension as well as adequate hydration during and following exercise is of greater concern. An exercise stress test may also be part of your medical evaluation to screen for ischemic heart changes (reduced blood flow during exercise due to blockages in the coronary arteries) or arrhythmias (abnormal heart rhythms) elicited by exercise. If cleared by your physician, you can safely participate in any activity. If a complication is detected, you can usually exercise safely within the limits of the complication, but you need to take special precautions as described for type 1 diabetic athletes (refer to chapter 5).

Appropriate Exercise Sessions

Any exercise should begin with an appropriate warm-up period consisting of 5 to 10 minutes of a low-level aerobic activity using the same muscles that will be exercised more intensely later in the workout. This active warm-up can take place before or after five to 10 minutes of static stretching. Following a period of higher-intensity activity, a cool-down period lasting five to 10 minutes should effectively bring the heart rate close to the preexercise level. (Refer to chapter 1 for a discussion of the usual components of an exercise session.)

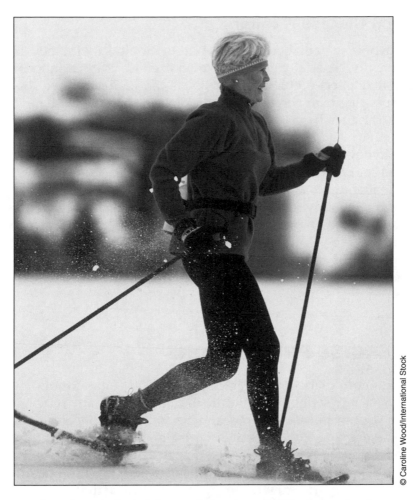

© Caroline Wood/International Stock

Any type of regular exercise training can help you control blood sugar levels.

Regular exercise training can have a beneficial effect on carbohydrate metabolism in people with type 2 diabetes. You should exercise according to the guidelines published by the ACSM (see chapter 1). In general, you should do an aerobic activity at a moderate intensity (60 to 90 percent of maximal heart rate) continuously for 20 to 60 minutes at a minimum of three to five days per week. The warm-up and cool-down periods are done in addition to the 20 to 60 minutes of more intense activity. Any physical activity, even if the activity is done at a lower level, can help control blood sugar levels in people with type 2 diabetes and is, therefore, highly recommended.

Blood Glucose Monitoring

All people with diabetes are advised to monitor their blood sugars frequently, especially before and after exercise. With monitoring, an activity's effect on blood sugar levels can be determined for each person. Regimen changes, mainly dietary changes for type 2 athletes, can then be made as needed to prevent hypoglycemia during an activity and even following it. People who use certain types of oral hypoglycemic medicines are at higher risk for developing low blood sugar levels. Type 2 athletes are not prone to developing ketosis (diabetic ketoacidosis) when blood sugar levels are high, which makes exercise with elevated blood sugar levels less dangerous for these people compared to people with type 1 diabetes. Knowing your starting blood sugar level, however, is important for implementation of appropriate regimen changes to prevent hypoglycemia and for maintaining proper hydration before, during, and after any physical activity.

EXERCISE PRECAUTIONS

People with diabetes who have good blood sugar control and do not have any serious complications can safely do any type of exercise. Most of the exercise precautions for type 1 diabetes apply almost equally to exercisers with type 2 diabetes, although the exercise issues for people with type 2 diabetes differ somewhat in a few areas. The following precautions apply to people with type 2 diabetes (not using insulin) who engage in physical activities.

Prevention of Hypoglycemia

Although less of a potential problem for type 2 athletes (compared with type 1 and other insulin users), prevention of hypoglycemia during physical activity is still a valid concern for type 2 diabetes. The incidence of low blood sugars resulting from exercise is generally low, however, unless these people are also taking certain oral medications and/or insulin injections. People who use certain oral hypoglycemic agents (such as Diabinese, DiaBeta, and Micronase) may be at higher risk for hypoglycemia than those who use other agents (refer to the discussion of the various oral hypoglycemic agents in chapter 3). If you begin exercise with blood sugars in a normal or near-normal range, especially if you use any of these medications, then you may need to consume additional carbohydrates to compensate for potential declines in blood sugars. You should use the general recommendations for diet changes alone for NPH or Lente users as a guide, even though you do not use insulin. When your blood sugars are already elevated at the start of an activity (in the range of 150 to 300 mg/dl or above), your risk of developing hypoglycemia during exercise is much lower, and you may not need any carbohydrate supplementation. If you use insulin, you should simply follow the recommendations given based on your insulin regimen and starting blood sugar levels. If you begin regular exercise training, reductions in your oral hypoglycemic agents and insulin may be necessary, but reductions should be made under the advice of a physician.

Prevention of Dehydration

Your risk for dehydration may be great if your blood sugars are not tightly controlled. Any elevation in blood sugars can cause a greater loss of water due to the increase in urination (polyuria). As a result, exercisers are especially at risk for dehydration when water loss through sweating adds to the level of dehydration. Exercise in the heat can be especially dangerous for these people, and adequate fluid replacement should be a high priority. Consume fluids before, during, and after exercise. Cool, plain water is the recommended beverage for fluid replacement. You should continue to drink extra fluids following all activity as it takes up to a day to fully restore fluids lost through sweat and ventilation.

Exercise With Complications

Diabetes-related complications are also a reality for many people with type 2 diabetes. They are susceptible to microvascular changes resulting from long-term diabetes such as nerve, eye, and kidney changes. Peripheral neuropathy (loss of feeling in feet and hands) is a common problem for type 2 people. Therefore, it may be best to avoid weight-bearing exercise if blisters or other potential damage could result from exercise and ultimately lead to a lower-limb amputation. Use precautionary measures for exercise involving the feet. Proper footwear is essential, especially for people with significant peripheral neuropathic changes. These people must closely monitor their feet for blisters and other damage both before and after exercise. Exercise with any microvascular conditions may require special precautions. These conditions include neuropathy (nerve disease), retinopathy (eye disease), and nephropathy (kidney disease). For a full discussion of these complications and exercise precautions, refer to chapter 5.

Heart disease. Diabetes accelerates the cardiovascular disease process. You have a higher risk for heart disease just by having diabetes, and your risk is greater if you have had diabetes longer than 10 years, have any other risk factors, evidence of microvascular changes, peripheral vascular disease, or nerve damage to your central nervous system (autonomic neuropathy). In these cases, you should undergo a graded exercise test under a physician's supervision before you embark on a moderate- or high-intensity exercise program. This exercise stress test will detect any significant coronary artery blockage or abnormal heart rhythms that may be worsened by exercise. Regular exercise can reduce insulin resistance, which is an important risk factor for premature heart disease in people with diabetes. Another potential benefit of exercise is a reduction in your heart disease risk by favorably altering elevated blood fats (cholesterol, triglycerides, HDL, and LDL) and coagulation defects along with lowering circulating insulin levels. The most consistent effect of regular exercise on lipids is a decrease in plasma triglyceride levels (circulating blood fats).

Hypertension. Elevations in blood pressure (hypertension) may also have long-term damaging effects on body systems. Hypertension is commonly associated with type 2 diabetes; both obesity and insulin resistance contribute to increases in blood pressure and may themselves result in chronical elevations. Regular exercise can lower body fat levels and reduce insulin resistance as well, resulting in modest decreases in both systolic (the higher blood pressure reading) and diastolic (the lower number) blood pressures. If you have hypertension, you must be more careful to avoid certain high-intensity or resistance exercises, which may cause blood pressure to rise to dangerously high levels during the activity. These activities may include heavy weight training; near-maximal exercise of any type; activities that require intense, sustained muscular contractions in the upper body such as water skiing or wind surfing; or exercises that require you to hold your breath (valsalva manuever).

Bobby Clarke

"He was skating on the cutting edge despite diabetes."

Robert Earle Clarke was first introduced to the ice rink at the age of three with a hockey stick in hand. Today, almost 50 years later, everyone knows him as "Bobby" Clarke, captain

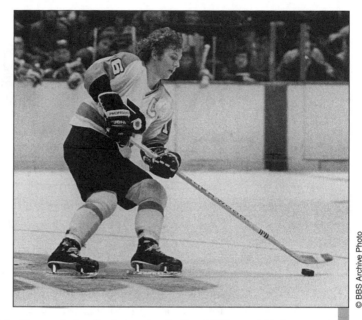

© BBS Archive Photo

of the Philadelphia Flyers during their heyday in the 1970s and their current president and general manager. Although he retired from active play and assumed managerial duties in 1985, he is still remembered as one of the Philadelphia Flyers's legendary Broad Street Bullies that gave Philadelphia its first and second Stanley Cup wins in their 1973-1974 and 1974-1975 seasons. He is still ranked as one of the Flyers's all-time offensive players during a 15-year professional career. In contrast to his rough reputation for play against other teams, he was a team player who often sacrificed his personal goal scoring for assists. He once said, "I'd just as soon set a goal up as get the goal."

His impressive hockey stat sheets do not reveal that Bobby was probably the first professional hockey player to have diabetes. His first question to his doctor when he was diagnosed with type 1 diabetes at the age of 13 was, "Will I be able to continue playing hockey?" Luckily, the doctor told him he would. Only twice in his hockey career did his blood sugars go dangerously low, requiring trips to the hospital. Early in his career, he did not like to discuss his diabetes with sports writers, who had a limited understanding of it. Some ignorant fans of opposing teams even taunted him by throwing packets of sugar and chocolate bars near him on the ice. Despite all this, he was among the first to use modern blood glucose testing devices. He remarked once that getting new technology first is one advantage of being in the athletic limelight.

Nowadays Bobby credits his good control to exercise. He runs 5 to 10 miles every morning, lifts weights, and uses in-line skates three times a week. He says, "I am a real firm believer in lots of exercise." He credits diabetes for educating him about nutrition. Early in his athletic career he learned how to manage carbohydrates for his exercise. While he says he does not eat a perfectly balanced diet with all the exchanges, he has a better diet than before he was diagnosed with diabetes.

EXERCISE BENEFITS

Despite the potential risks associated with exercise, the benefits to people with type 2 diabetes generally far outweigh the risks (see chapter 1 for a list of all the benefits). Think of your diabetes as a reminder to take better care of yourself, to eat right, and to exercise daily. Find a way to exercise as much as you are capable of doing, because it can only help improve your diabetes control and prevent long-term health problems. *Any physical activity, no matter how minor, is better than none in helping to lessen your insulin resistance, lower your body fat, and maintain your metabolically active muscle mass.* When you begin exercise at an early age, you can delay or even prevent the onset of type 2 diabetes. When exercise is begun in the early stage of diabetes (when only insulin resistance and slight increases in blood sugar levels may be evident), the full onset of type 2 diabetes can actually be delayed or prevented. Follow the basic guidelines discussed in this chapter and monitor your own body's response. Use frequent blood sugar monitoring to learn the effects of different types and amounts of exercise.

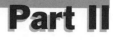

Part II

Sports
and
Fitness
Activities

Chapter 7

Endurance Sports

So do you want to run a marathon, cycle up a mountain, or compete in a full Ironman triathlon? Athletes with diabetes have done all these things and more! Their examples, as well as other examples relevant to the more modest athlete, are included in this chapter. The following activities are included: running and jogging, marathons, cross country running, soccer, cross-country skiing, rowing, swimming, cycling, triathlons, and ultraendurance events and training.

Endurance sports generally stress the aerobic energy system. Energy in the form of ATP can be produced from carbohydrate, fat, and protein sources utilizing this system. In general, the intensity and duration of an activity largely determine the fuels used. Less intense activities such as slow swimming may use a greater amount of circulating blood fats (free fatty acids) along with some muscular stores of triglycerides (storage form of fat), muscle glycogen, and blood glucose. Moderate to intense activities use a greater amount of carbohydrate, mainly muscle glycogen, and also blood glucose sources. Very intense efforts use carbohydrate sources almost exclusively. Very prolonged activities such as marathoning potentially use more fat as well as protein stores (up to 10 to 15 percent of the total energy) as muscle and liver glycogen stores become depleted. The lactic acid system may be used during an aerobic activity whenever the pace is increased or faster muscle fibers are recruited. You can generally delay fatigue during prolonged bouts of endurance exercise by ingesting carbohydrates during the activity. Ingesting rapidly-absorbed carbohydrate may be especially important in maintaining blood sugar levels during a sustained activity. For a fuller explanation of the various energy systems and energy sources used for different types of exercise, refer to chapter 2.

This chapter covers general recommendations for endurance sports. Then within the discussion of each endurance activity, both general recommendations and real-life examples of some athletes' specific changes in insulin and diet are listed according to their insulin regimen (NPH and Lente, insulin pump, and Ultralente users). *Users of oral hypoglycemic agents are not listed separately, but the general recommendations under diet changes alone (or specifically for NPH and Lente users, if given by insulin regimen) can be used as an approximate guide for type 2 diabetic people when blood sugars at the start of or during exercise are in a normal range.* However, when your blood sugars are elevated, you are less likely to need increased carbohydrate intake. After embarking on your regular endurance exercise program, it is likely that you will have to lower your doses of prescribed medicines. However, you should only make reductions in oral doses of medication under the advice of your physician. For more information about the actions of various types of insulins or oral hypoglycemic agents, refer to chapter 3.

GENERAL RECOMMENDATIONS

The commonality of endurance sports is their use of the aerobic energy system to provide fuels for these longer-duration activities. In general, the more intense the activity is, the more you rely on carbohydrate as the primary fuel source. Although muscle glycogen provides a much greater proportion of the total carbohydrate used, the blood glucose supply becomes more important when glycogen stores become depleted, when insulin levels are high, when blood sugar levels are high, or when the exercising person is untrained. Ingesting an adequate amount of carbohydrate to counteract the muscles' use of blood glucose is essential in preventing hypoglycemia during exercise.

General Diet and Insulin Changes

Prolonged activities require greater reductions in insulin doses (see table 7.1). While more fat may be used as a fuel along with carbohydrate for slower and longer activities, glycogen stores will also be depleted more by the end of the activity, which ultimately leads to a greater reliance on the use of blood glucose to finish the exercise. In especially prolonged activities, a combination of both insulin changes and food changes is usually necessary to maintain blood sugar levels. If you do an activity when circulating insulin levels are lower, such as three to four hours following your last dose of short-acting insulin, then you may not need to make as many changes in your insulin dosage. In these cases, you can either ingest extra carbohydrate or make no changes for blood sugar maintenance.

In general, you may need a carbohydrate supplementation of 15 to 45 grams for every 30 to 60 minutes of a prolonged activity depending on the intensity and duration. You can best determine your need for carbohydrate by measuring your blood sugar responses during the exercise. You will need more carbohydrates when you exercise during a peak of either short-acting insulin or NPH or Lente if you do not sufficiently reduce insulin doses. You may need additional food at the end of an activity and even at bedtime to prevent a drop in blood sugar later as glycogen stores are being replaced, especially following a prolonged activity.

Your carbohydrate requirement is not as great with shorter, more intense activities as it is with lower-intensity, more prolonged activities (see table 7.2). Although you use a greater percentage of carbohydrate to fuel these shorter, intense activities, their intensity causes a larger release of hormones that raise blood glucose, and blood sugars are more effectively maintained during shorter, intense

Table 7.1 **General Insulin Reductions for Endurance Sports**[a]

Duration	Low-intensity	Moderate-intensity	High-intensity
		Insulin reductions[b]	
15 min	none	5-10%	0-15%[c]
30 min	none	10-20%	10-30%
45 min	5-15%	15-30%	20-45%
60 min	10-20%	20-40%	30-60%
90 min	15-30%	30-55%	45-75%
120 min	20-40%	40-70%	60-90%
180 min	30-60%	60-90%	75-100%

[a]These insulin recommendations assume that no additional food is eaten before or during the activity to compensate. For insulin pump users, basal rate reductions during an activity may be greater or lesser than these recommendations, and they may be done alone or along with reduced bolus amounts.

[b]These insulin reductions apply to the specific insulin peaking during exercise (Regular or Humalog for an activity following a meal, or morning NPH or Lente during afternoon exercise). A lesser insulin reduction may be needed if exercise occurs more than 3 to 4 hours following the last injection of short-acting insulin. Postexercise insulin reductions may also be necessary.

[c]For intense, near-maximal exercise, an actual increase in short-acting insulin (rather than a decrease) may be necessary to counter the glucose-raising effects of hormones released during exercise.

Table 7.2   **General Carbohydrate Increases for Endurance Sports**[a]

Duration	Intensity[b]	Blood sugar prior to exercise (mg/dl)			
		<100	100-150	150-200	>200[c]
	Low	0-5	none	none	none
15 min	Moderate	5-10	0-10	0-5	none
	High[d]	0-15	0-15	0-10	0-5
	Low	5-10	0-10	none	none
30 min	Moderate	10-25	10-20	5-15	0-10
	High	15-35	15-30	10-25	5-20
	Low	5-15	5-10	0-5	none
45 min	Moderate	15-35	10-30	5-20	0-10
	High	20-40	20-35	15-30	10-25
	Low	10-15	10-15	5-10	0-5
60 min	Moderate	20-50	15-40	10-30	5-15
	High	30-45	25-40	20-35	15-30
	Low	15-20	10-20	5-15	0-10
90 min	Moderate	30-60	25-50	20-35	10-20
	High	45-70	40-60	30-50	25-40
	Low	15-30	15-25	10-20	5-15
120 min	Moderate	40-80	35-70	30-50	15-30
	High	60-90	50-80	40-70	30-60
	Low	30-45	25-40	20-30	10-20
180 min	Moderate	60-120	50-100	40-80	25-45
	High	90-135	75-120	60-105	45-90

[a]The recommended quantity is given in grams of rapidly absorbed carbohydrate. One fruit or one bread exchange equals 15 grams of carbohydrate.

[b]Low-intensity activities are done at less than 50%, moderate activities at 50-70%, and high-intensity activities at 70-85% of heart rate reserve (refer to chapter 1).

[c]For blood sugars above this level, or when ketones are present, an additional dose of short-acting insulin may be required to reduce these levels during an activity, and the recommended carbohydrate intake may be higher than actually needed.

[d]Intense (near-maximal), short-duration exercise may actually cause blood sugar levels to increase.

activities. Obviously, greater reductions in insulin decrease the need for extra carbohydrates.

NPH and Lente users. Some reductions in insulin doses will depend on whether you take the NPH or Lente in the morning and evening or just at bedtime. If you take short-acting insulin alone during the day, you can reduce preworkout doses by 10 to 75 percent when the activity follows a meal, depending on the expected length and intensity of the exercise and increase in carbohydrate intake. Morning NPH or Lente users may need to reduce those insulin doses by 10 to 50 percent for a planned or continuing activity in the afternoon. If you exercise when circulating insulin levels are lower, such as three to four hours following the last injection of short-acting insulin (when you take NPH at bedtime only), then you may need minimal insulin changes, and you can eat extra carbohydrate if necessary. Following prolonged endurance exercise, you may need to reduce insulin for meals by 25 to 50 percent, and you may reduce bedtime doses of NPH or Lente by a small amount (10 to 30 percent) as well to prevent nocturnal hypoglycemia if you do not increase your carbohydrate intake.

Insulin pump users. If you are a pump user, you may lower your basal insulin infusion rate during an activity by 0 to 100 percent, depending on the intensity and duration of the exercise and how much extra carbohydrate you wish to supplement. In addition, you can reduce preworkout meal boluses by 10 to 75 percent if exercise follows closely after the meal, depending on your intake of extra carbohydrate. If you do an activity when circulating insulin levels are lower, such as three to four hours following your last insulin bolus, then you may not need as much change in insulin doses or food intake. Following prolonged endurance exercise, you may need to reduce insulin boluses for meals by 25 to 50 percent. You may need to reduce basal rates of insulin by a small amount (10 to 25 percent) as well for a period of time (usually 2 to 6 hours, but up to 24) following the activity to prevent later-onset and nocturnal hypoglycemia.

Ultralente users. For endurance activities, you can reduce preworkout doses of short-acting insulin by 10 to 75 percent when the activity follows a meal, depending on the expected length and intensity of the exercise and increase in carbohydrate intake. You may need to reduce your morning dose of Ultralente by 10 to 30 percent for an activity continuing into the late afternoon. If you exercise when

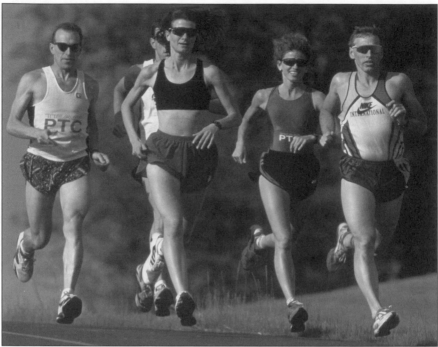

© Greg Crisp/SportsChrome USA

Prolonged running requires using substantial amounts of muscle glycogen and blood glucose as fuel. You may need to increase your carbohydrate intake and lower your insulin doses to compensate.

circulating insulin levels are lower, such as three to four hours following your last injection of short-acting insulin, then you may need minimal insulin changes or extra carbohydrate. Following prolonged endurance exercise, you may need to reduce insulin for meals by 25 to 50 percent, reduce bedtime doses of Ultralente by a small amount (10 to 20 percent) to prevent nocturnal hypoglycemia, and eat extra carbohydrate.

Intensity, Duration, and Other Effects

Many variables can affect blood sugar response to an endurance activity. The intensity and duration of the activity will have a significant impact on blood sugars; in general, more intense activities done for a shorter period of time will result in a smaller drop in blood sugars compared with prolonged, slower activities. Circulating insulin levels during the activity will also have an effect on your blood sugar. Exercise early in the morning (especially before you inject any insulin) may require substantially fewer regimen changes than activities later in the day when insulin levels are higher. Depending on the insulin regimen, circulating levels can also be low during exercise, resulting in a lesser or minimal need for carbohydrate supplementation. Your starting blood sugar levels will also affect your need for regimen changes: you need fewer changes when blood sugar levels start in a higher range. Also, your basal insulin needs may be lower with regular endurance training, resulting in lower doses of all insulins regardless of the specific insulin regimen you follow.

RUNNING AND JOGGING

These activities are very aerobic in nature as they stress endurance. The main fuels used by the body are fat and carbohydrate, with carbohydrate use (both blood glucose and muscle glycogen) increasing with running intensity.

Running intensity, duration, time of day that you run, circulating insulin levels, and starting blood sugar levels have the biggest effects on blood sugar response. Exercise intensity will affect the release of glucose-raising hormones, with more intense running resulting in a possible increase in blood sugar levels (e.g., intense 5K races or sprint and interval training). The longer the duration of the run, the more energy is provided by stores of muscle and liver glycogen, making it harder to maintain blood sugar levels for prolonged runs without carbohydrate supplementation. Using more muscle glycogen will increase insulin sensitivity following the exercise, increasing the risk for later-onset hypoglycemia. Circulating insulin levels will also affect the need for carbohydrate supplementation. If you run when circulating insulin levels are lower (generally before meals for all insulin regimens, except before lunch for morning NPH or Lente users), exercise will not cause blood sugars to drop as much because the body's response is more normal due to the lower insulin levels. Pump users can most easily create normal amounts of insulin during exercise by suspending basal insulin rates. Insulin levels are often low early in the morning for all insulin users, and at that time, insulin resistance is greatest. Therefore, if you run before breakfast, you will have more stable blood sugar levels with less need for extra carbohydrate. If blood sugars are higher in the morning, you may need a small dose of short-acting insulin to prevent a rise in blood sugars by the end of the run. Higher blood sugars at a

RUNNING AND JOGGING

User	Insulin	Diet
NPH/Lente	• For shorter runs following a meal, reduce short-acting insulin doses by 10-30% (especially if NPH or Lente doses are taken at bedtime only). • For afternoon runs, reduce the morning dose of NPH/Lente (if taken) by 10-20%. • For longer runs, reduce insulin even more (20-50%). • For early-morning running before an insulin dose, no insulin or diet changes may be necessary due to the low circulating levels of insulin and high insulin resistance at that time of day. • For higher starting blood sugars, an additional injection of short-acting insulin (0.5-3 units) may be necessary to prevent further increases in blood sugars resulting from the run, especially early in the morning. • Consider decreasing the dosage of short-acting insulins by 10-30% for the meal following a run, or compensate with extra carbohydrate. • Reduce bedtime doses of NPH or Lente by 10-20%, or eat a bedtime snack to prevent nocturnal hypoglycemia, especially if a run is longer or unusual.	• Supplementing with 10-20 grams of carbohydrate may be necessary, based on starting blood sugar levels and insulin reductions for shorter runs. • If circulating insulin levels are low at the start of exercise (i.e., 3-4 hours after the last injection of short-acting insulin if you take NPH at bedtime only), eat less carbohydrate. • A longer morning run (more than 45 minutes) may require some extra food after the initial 15-30 minutes of running. With a starting blood sugar of 200 mg/dl, no extra carbohydrate may be necessary for most runs at any time of day. • Eat an additional snack of about 15 grams of carbohydrate for shorter afternoon runs if morning NPH or lunchtime short-acting insulin is not reduced by at least 10-20%. • For every 30-45 minutes of running, 10-20 grams of carbohydrate may be necessary for longer runs. • More intense running (road races or interval training) usually requires less supplementation due to a greater release of glucose-raising hormones, especially when done in the morning.
Insulin Pump	• Decrease or discontinue basal insulin rates during runs. • For shorter runs of 3 miles or less, suspend the pump altogether to provide a more normal insulin response to exercise. Doing so usually eliminates the need for extra carbohydrate. • Reduce boluses by 10-30% for meals before and following the run to prevent low blood sugars, depending on changes in basal rates and carbohydrate intake.	• Consider consuming an extra 10-20 grams of carbohydrate every 30-45 minutes for long runs. • If basal rates are not reduced for shorter runs, supplement with 15-30 grams of carbohydrate. • For runs of any length early in the morning before a meal bolus (especially intense running such as road races or interval training), minimal carbohydrate supplementation may be necessary, and basal insulin rates may need to be reduced less.

User	Insulin	Diet
Insulin Pump	• For longer runs, reducing the basal rates by 50-100% during the run as well as preexercise boluses will help maintain blood sugar levels. • Basal rates may need to remain low for several hours following the exercise (or even overnight) for especially long or unusual runs. • For higher starting blood sugars, an additional injection of short-acting insulin (0.5-3 units) may be necessary to prevent further increases in blood sugars.	• With a starting blood sugar of 200 mg/dl, consume no extra food for shorter runs or during the first 30 minutes of longer runs.
Ultralente	• Reduce short-acting insulin by 10-30% for the meal before exercise (within 2-3 hours) for shorter runs (or 20-50% for longer ones) to prevent low blood sugars during a run. • For the meal following exercise, consider reducing short-acting insulin by 10-30% also. • For preplanned longer runs, reduce morning doses of Ultralente by 10-20% to prevent postexercise hypoglycemia later in the day, or eat additional snacks after running. • For higher starting blood sugars, an additional injection of insulin (0.5-3 units) may be necessary to prevent further increases in blood sugars resulting from the run.	• Exercising with reduced basal circulating insulin levels (at least 2-3 hours after a Humalog or 3-4 hours after a regular insulin dose) minimizes the need for carbohydrate supplementation, at least for shorter runs of 3 miles or less. • Eat an additional 10-20 grams of carbohydrate per 30-45 minutes of running. • For runs of any length early in the morning before breakfast, very little carbohydrate supplementation may be necessary. • A longer run of more than 45 minutes may require some extra food after the initial 30 minutes of running, depending on the blood sugar response. • With a starting blood sugar of 200 mg/dl or less, consume no extra carbohydrate initially. • More intense running (road races or interval training) usually requires less supplementation to maintain blood sugars, especially when done in the morning.

later time of day may require less of an adjustment as running will usually cause blood sugar to drop.

Athlete Examples

In real life, diabetic athletes use every combination of insulin and diet changes to compensate for running, depending on a number of different factors. If weight loss is a goal, then insulin changes alone may be most preferred.

Insulin Changes Alone

An NPH user reduces his prebreakfast NPH by 1 unit (from 6 to 5 units) when he runs intensely for up to two hours in the afternoon. For morning runs, he reduces his regular prebreakfast insulin by 1 unit (from 4 to 3 units). He finds that running generally causes his blood sugars to drop, but that they actually increase when he runs intense, short (5K) races that take about 16 minutes.

A pump user runs five to 10 miles (about an 8-minute mile pace) and reduces the basal dosage on her pump to 0.3 units per hour (from 0.5) unless she is running uphill or at higher altitude; then she reduces the basal to 0.1 or 0.2 units per hour.

Diet Changes Alone

A Lente user usually runs 3.5 to 5 miles early in the morning without changing his Lente dose. He tries to eat 125 to 150 calories worth of carbohydrates (including half a banana and a quarter of a bagel) and hydrate well before the exercise. If his starting blood sugar is near 200 mg/dl, he will not eat anything. If it is more than 200, he takes 1 to 3 units of Humalog before exercising. Starting at much less than 140 mg/dl impairs his workout.

Combined Insulin and Diet Changes

An NPH user runs six to seven days a week, usually between 5 and 8 miles. If he runs before lunch, he makes sure that his blood sugar levels are at least 90 mg/dl, eats one-third of a PowerBar for every 25 to 30 minutes of running, and eats lunch when finished. If he runs early in the morning, he will eat PowerBars only as needed during his run, then take his insulin and eat breakfast afterward. If he runs in the evening before dinner, he takes Regular insulin to cover his dinner after the run, adjusting his dose down based on the length of his run. He has noticed that with shorter races (5K), his blood sugar levels actually go up after a hard effort.

A pump user reduces the amount of insulin circulating in his body at the time of exercise by reducing his pump basal rate from 0.7 units per hour to 0.4 starting two to three hours before running. If he eats before running, he tries to eat at least two hours before and takes a Humalog bolus of no more than 1.5 units. If he runs immediately after eating, he does not take a meal bolus, but he will take a reduced bolus after the exercise. He determines his carbohydrate intake during his run by his blood sugars. For early morning runs when he is more insulin resistant, he reduces his basal less (to 0.5) or not at all and balances as he needs to with carbohydrate intake.

For sprint training after dinner, an Ultralente user takes 1 unit less of her morning Ultralente dose and 1 to 2 units less of her immediately preceding short-acting insulin and consumes more carbohydrates (dates, prunes, and Fig Newtons).

For normal runs after breakfast, another Ultralente user will eat 15 to 30 extra grams of carbohydrate at breakfast. When he runs in the afternoon, he supplements the same way but if his sugars are 200 mg/dl or above, he eats nothing. For longer runs of 10 miles or more, he reduces his Ultralente dose by 1 to 2 units in the morning.

Intensity, Duration, and Other Effects

Effect of previous days of exercise. An NPH user varies his regimen based on his previous days of exercise. On the first day of running 30 minutes in the morning (after one or more days of rest), he makes no immediate adjustments to his morning insulin (usually 2 units of Humalog and 10 units of NPH), but he may cut his Humalog by 1 unit at dinner and his NPH by 1 unit at bedtime. On the second day, he reduces his morning dosage by 1 unit of Humalog and 1 unit of NPH, with similar dinner and bedtime adjustments. On the third day in a row, he reduces his morning dose by 2 units each and also reduces his dinner and bedtime doses by 1 to 2 units and increases his carbohydrate intake during the day and at bedtime.

Effect of time of day (early morning). An Ultralente user usually runs for 45 minutes before breakfast. If her fasting blood sugar is 160 to 260 mg/dl, she takes her usual morning dose of Humalog, waits 15 minutes, and then exercises without eating because her morning blood sugars in that range are resistant to change. If her blood sugar is below 160, she runs and then takes 20 percent less Humalog with her breakfast. If her blood sugar is below 80 mg/dl, she will drink four ounces of orange juice before exercising.

Effect of exercise intensity and seasonal training. An Ultralente user runs 5K races competitively. He trains six days a week for nine months of the year, alternating moderate-intensity days with high-intensity workouts. During the hard part of his training season, he permanently decreases his Ultralente doses (morning and evening) from 15 units to 13 or 14. He adds 15 to 30 grams of carbohydrate snacks before exercise, ingests one glucose tablet (4 grams of carbohydrate) every five minutes during his workout, and adds extra calories from all sources to his diet throughout the day on his more active days. For his high-intensity workouts, he does not need to eat as much carbohydrate before, but he finds that he needs to eat twice as much food after and decrease his Ultralente dose by 1 unit. For competitions he does not need to take any supplemental carbohydrates if his starting blood sugar is above 120 mg/dl. If below, he adds 15 to 30 grams of carbohydrate 30 minutes before the race. He always experiences an increase in his blood sugar during races due to the maximal effort. Before races he takes 50 percent of his usual morning dose of Humalog to prevent large increases in blood sugar.

MARATHONS

Participation in marathons involves high-mileage training as well as covering the distance of 26.2 miles at maximal race pace. This activity is almost purely aerobic in nature, resulting in significant depletion of muscle glycogen in many different muscles due to its prolonged duration. The body's main fuels are carbohydrate and fat, and carbohydrate use (both blood glucose and muscle glycogen) increases even more for greater running intensities. While the choice remains to alter insulin doses or carbohydrate intake, marathoning usually requires a combination of the two due to its prolonged nature, regardless of the athlete's insulin regimen. Prevention of fatigue during a marathon run requires the intake of additional carbohydrate to help maintain blood glucose levels. The

MARATHONS

User	Insulin	Diet
NPH/Lente	• Consider reducing pre-event evening NPH or Lente doses by as much as 50%, but expect that doing so will result in higher blood sugar levels prior to the event. • Reduce prebreakfast NPH or Lente by 25-50% before running, and reduce short-acting insulin dose by 25-75%, depending on fasting blood sugar levels. • Postrun meals may require a smaller dose of short-acting insulin for a given amount of carbohydrate while insulin sensitivity remains heightened. • Reduce evening NPH or Lente dose by 10-30% to prevent nocturnal hypoglycemia, especially if marathon-length runs are an unusual activity.	• Supplement with 15-30 grams of carbohydrate for every 30-45 minutes of exercise, depending on blood sugar levels. • Starting with a higher blood sugar will usually require less supplementation, at least during the early stages of the run.
Insulin Pump	• Do not alter basal insulin rates until the morning of the race, but reduce basal rate during the event by 25-100% to minimize circulating levels of insulin. • Reduce boluses for prerun meals by 25-75% depending on fasting blood sugar levels. • Reduce boluses for meals later in the day by 25-50% depending on blood sugar readings. • Due to the possibility of post-exercise late-onset hypoglycemia, basal rates during the rest of the day and the following night may also remain 10-25% lower.	• Supplement with 15-30 grams of carbohydrate for every 30-60 minutes of exercise, depending on blood sugar levels and the reduction in basal insulin rates. • Starting with a higher blood sugar will usually require less supplementation (at least initially) during the run.
Ultralente	• Circulating insulin levels at the start of the marathon can be minimized with a 10-25% reduction in the previous evening's Ultralente dose, if desired. • Reduce morning short-acting insulin doses for any food eaten before the event by 25-75%, depending on fasting blood sugar levels.	• Supplement with 15-30 grams of carbohydrate for every 30-60 minutes of exercise, depending on blood sugar levels. • Starting a marathon with a higher blood sugar will usually require less supplementation, at least initially, during the run.

(continued)

MARATHONS *(continued)*

User	Insulin	Diet
Ultralente	• Reduce the morning Ultralente dose before the event by 10-50% if you take Ultralente twice a day. • Reduce the evening dose of Ultralente to a lesser extent (10-25%). The amount of the reduction depends on the reduction in the morning dose (i.e., a greater reduction in the morning dose may require a lesser or no reduction of the evening dose). • Reduce doses of short-acting insulin following the event by 25-50%, depending on blood sugar readings and carbohydrate intake during the race.	

actual changes you make will depend on factors such as blood sugar and circulating insulin levels at the beginning of the marathon run.

The key to maintaining blood sugar levels during a marathon is minimizing the levels of circulating insulin during the event by decreasing NPH, Lente, or Ultralente doses the evening before the race and/or reducing or eliminating meal boluses before running. Pump users can most easily minimize circulating insulin levels by decreasing basal insulin rates just before and during the race.

Athlete Examples

Diabetic marathoners have tried a variety of strategies to maximize their performances during the event. All of their regimen changes involve decreases in insulin and increases in carbohydrate intake.

Combined Insulin and Diet Changes

For half marathons at a 9- to 10-minute mile pace, an NPH user takes only half of her usual morning dose of NPH. If her blood sugar is less than 100 mg/dl, she eats two bananas. If it is 120 to 150, she eats one banana. She rechecks her blood sugar after six miles and supplements with a carbohydrate drink or with 1 to 2 units of Humalog, in order to keep her blood sugar between 100 and 120 during the race.

For half or full marathons, a Lente user reduces his nightly Lente dose by as much as 50 percent as well as his premeal Humalog by 80 percent (from his usual 10 units to 2) and consumes gels, dextrose, and sport bars during the competition as needed. He tries to keep his blood sugar around 200 mg/dl during competitions and workouts.

For a marathon, an insulin pump user makes adjustments based on her starting blood sugar. If her blood sugar is less than 120 mg/dl, she reduces her basal rate during the run from 0.7 units per hour to 0.3 units per hour. She also eats a banana before running. For blood sugar between 120 and 200, she modifies her basal insulin the same way, but she does not eat any extra food. For blood sugar higher than 200 mg/dl, she reduces the basal rate to only 0.4 units per hour and does not eat a snack. She carries a diluted sport drink with her and takes three to four swallows from it every five minutes during the run, and she eats a Power Gel halfway through her run.

One Ultralente user finds that the key to maintaining blood sugar levels during a marathon is to not inject any Humalog in the morning before running a half marathon. She eats 20 grams of carbohydrate just before the run without taking any Humalog. She also reduces her Ultralente dose the night before as well as the morning of the race by 50 percent. During the race she drinks a diluted sport drink and carries glucose tablets with her. She eats carbohydrates after the race and doses with Humalog according to her blood sugar readings.

For marathons, another Ultralente user takes 3 to 4 units of Regular only and no Humalog (he usually takes 4 units each of Humalog and Regular insulin), but he does not adjust his Ultralente dose. He tries to begin a race with his blood sugar between 150 and 200 mg/dl, and then he supplements with PowerBars during the event, eating half of a bar every 30 minutes. After exercise he uses Regular insulin instead of Humalog because it gets into his system a lot more slowly.

CROSS COUNTRY RUNNING

This sport is very aerobic in nature as it exclusively stresses endurance performance. Carbohydrate use (both blood glucose and muscle glycogen) increases with running intensity; actual responses will vary with the duration of running as well as the intensity. With any insulin regimen, the choice is to alter insulin doses, diet, or both, depending on other factors such as the time of day you exercise, blood sugar levels, and circulating insulin levels during exercise.

The intensity and duration of running can have a significant impact on blood sugar response. In general, more intense running (such as for competitions) will result in a decreased drop in blood sugar than more prolonged, slower runs. The circulating insulin levels during the activity will also have an effect. With the insulin pump or Ultralente insulin regimens, circulating levels can be quite low during exercise, which reduces the need for carbohydrate supplementation. In addition, basal insulin needs may be lower overall during the cross country season, requiring lower doses of all insulins regardless of which specific insulin regimen you follow.

Athlete Examples

These examples show the variety of insulin and carbohydrate modifications that you can use for cross country running as well as the effects of exercise intensity.

Diet Changes Alone

For one- to two-hour cross country runs up to 16 miles, an NPH user tries to start with his blood sugar between 90 and 140 mg/dl, then eats one-third of a PowerBar for every 25 to 30 minutes of running. He tends to eat a lot after he finishes his run.

Combined Insulin and Diet Changes

An NPH user runs 4 miles in the mornings and 6 to 10 miles in the afternoon most days of the week for cross country practice. For this activity, he cuts his NPH dose in half in the morning on practice days and supplements with a food bar such as granola bars, 64 ounces of a sport drink, and two PowerBars.

Intensity, Duration, and Other Effects

Effect of exercise intensity. An Ultralente user participates in cross country practices that involve 40 to 60 minutes of continuous running, followed by sprints at the end of practice. If she has low

CROSS COUNTRY RUNNING

User	Insulin	Diet
NPH/Lente*	• Reduce morning doses of NPH or Lente by 10-50% for planned afternoon practices. • If only short-acting insulin is taken during the day, reduce the preworkout bolus by 10-30% depending on the expected length and intensity of practice. • If the practice is more than 3-4 hours following the last injection of insulin, then make minimal reductions in insulin. • For morning meets, when running is shorter and more intense, reduce precompetition short-acting insulin by 10-30% without making changes in morning NPH doses. • Reduce NPH or Lente doses during the cross country training season by up to 10-30%.	• For afternoon practices, eat an additional 15-30 grams of carbohydrate for every 30 minutes of running, especially if you do not reduce morning NPH doses. • The greater the prior reduction in insulin doses, the smaller the food supplementation will need to be. • Eat additional carbohydrate at the end of practice to prevent hypoglycemia, especially for longer practices. • For morning meets or competitions, eat fewer supplemental carbohydrates as early-morning insulin resistance will keep blood sugars more level.
Insulin Pump	• Reduce basal insulin infusion rate during a practice or competition by 25-100% depending on the amount of additional carbohydrate eaten. • Reduce prepractice meal boluses by 25-50% for exercise closely following a meal. • For morning meets (involving shorter and more intense runs), consider reducing precompetition short-acting insulin by 10-30%. • Reduce basal rates overall during the cross country training season by 10-25%.	• Eat 15-30 grams of carbohydrate for every 30 minutes of running, depending on insulin reductions and the initial blood sugar level. • More intense running (competitions), especially in the morning when insulin resistance is higher, may require less supplementation due to a greater release of glucose-raising hormones.
Ultralente	• For regular practices, reduce short-acting insulin dose before exercise by 25-50% to reduce the need for extra carbohydrate. • For morning meets (involving shorter and more intense runs), precompetition short-acting insulins will need to be reduced by 10-30%. • Reduce Ultralente doses by 10-25% during the cross-country season compared with the off-season.	• Eat an extra 15-30 grams of carbohydrate for every 30 minutes of running, depending on the blood sugar level at the beginning of exercise and length of time since the last injection of short-acting insulin. • More intense running (competitions), especially in the morning when insulin resistance is higher, may require less supplementation due to a greater release of glucose-raising hormones.

* Reductions in insulin doses will depend on whether the NPH or Lente is taken in the morning and evening, or just at bedtime.

blood sugar, she will have a granola bar, juice, or sport drink. Before a cross country race (2 miles), if her blood sugar is more than 150 mg/dl, she will take 1 unit of Humalog for every 50 mg/dl of excess blood sugar; otherwise, her blood sugar goes too high when she races.

SOCCER

Depending on the position you play, this activity is a combination of stop-and-start movements, power moves such as kicking or throwing the ball, and longer runs. Midfielders (halfbacks) may do more sustained running, whereas fullbacks and goalies may run only in short bursts. You will need changes in both insulin and carbohydrate intake for most soccer play. Changes will vary with the position you play and the duration of the activity. However, if no insulin changes are made for soccer games and practices, supplementation with additional carbohydrate (30 to 45 grams per hour) will be needed for all insulin regimens, depending on the levels of circulating insulin and the intensity and duration of the play.

Intensity (often determined by the position played), duration of play, and levels of circulating insulin at the time of play are the factors that affect the blood sugar response to soccer. Prolonged play will cause greater reductions in muscle glycogen stores and blood sugar levels and will require greater carbohydrate intake combined with reductions in insulin both before and possibly after playing. The position you play (whether it involves fairly continuous running or just occasional action) largely determines the intensity of play. A midfielder (halfback) running more continuously for an hour-long game will need to reduce insulin and increase food intake much more than a goalie, who occasionally kicks or throws the ball without running much. During practices, activity levels among positions may be more similar if all team members do continuous running or shooting drills. The level of circulating insulin during play will also affect the need for carbohydrate supplementation. If you have taken short-acting insulins within three to four hours of the activity, glucose levels are more likely to drop than if only basal amounts of insulin are present in your body during soccer play. During the soccer season, you will probably need to reduce basal insulin doses (intermediate and long-acting insulins or a pump basal rate) more than during off-season times.

SOCCER

User	Insulin	Diet
NPH/Lente	• For morning soccer, reduce short-acting insulin doses before breakfast by 10-30%. • For soccer practices and games in the afternoon, reduce morning doses of NPH or Lente by 10-30% or reduce lunchtime short-acting insulin doses by 15-40%. • For soccer later in the afternoon, smaller changes may be necessary due to lower circulating levels of insulin at that time of day. • Following prolonged or intense soccer, reduce doses of short-acting insulin for meals by 20-30%, and reduce evening doses of NPH or Lente by 10-30% as well.	• Supplement with 15-30 grams of carbohydrate per hour for soccer play, depending on reductions in insulin and the intensity and duration of play. • More carbohydrate after intense, prolonged play and an additional bedtime snack may also be necessary to prevent hypoglycemia later or overnight.
Insulin Pump	• During any soccer play, reduce basal rates on the insulin pump by 25-100% depending on the length and intensity of play. • A midfielder running more continuously for an hour-long game may need a reduction of 50-75% compared with a goalie (25%). • For morning play, reduce breakfast doses of short-acting insulin by 10-30% depending on reductions in basal rate during the activity. • For soccer practices and games in the afternoon, reduce lunchtime insulin boluses by 20-30% if playing within 3-4 hours of the injection. • If playing more than 3-4 hours afterward, reduced basal rates and/or extra food may suffice. • Following prolonged or intense play, reduce insulin boluses for the next meal by 20-30% as well as overnight basal insulin rates by 10-25% unless an additional bedtime snack is eaten.	• Eat 15-30 grams of additional carbohydrate per hour for soccer play, depending on reductions in insulin basal rates and boluses and the intensity and duration of play. • More carbohydrate after intense, prolonged play and an additional bedtime snack may also be necessary to prevent hypoglycemia from occurring.
Ultralente	• For morning practices and games, reduce breakfast doses of short-acting insulin by 10-30%.	• Eat 15-30 grams of additional carbohydrate per hour for practices or afternoon games, depending on the

(continued)

SOCCER (continued)

User	Insulin	Diet
Ultralente	• For soccer practices and games in the afternoon, decrease lunchtime doses of short-acting insulin by 20-30% if exercise occurs within 3-4 hours of dosage. • Following prolonged or intense soccer play, reduce short-acting insulin doses for the next meal by 20-30% as well as evening Ultralente doses by 10-20%, or eat an additional bedtime snack. • If you exercise more than 3-4 hours after the last injection of short-acting insulin, you may need smaller regimen changes to compensate.	reductions in insulin and the intensity and duration of play. • Eat extra carbohydrate after intense, prolonged play and possibly an additional bedtime snack to prevent later-onset hypoglycemia.

Athlete Examples

These examples mainly show combined insulin and diet changes to compensate for soccer play. If you are concerned about weight loss resulting from soccer play, you should rely on supplemental carbohydrates more heavily to increase caloric intake.

Combined Insulin and Diet Changes

On the afternoons that an NPH user has soccer practice, he does not make any adjustments before his activity, but he decreases his dinner Humalog by 1 unit following practice or games. He keeps juice, regular soda, glucose tablets, and candy available to treat low blood sugars. If his blood sugar is below 90 mg/dl at bedtime, he eats an additional carbohydrate (15 grams) and a protein with his bedtime snack.

Another NPH user participates in two-hour soccer practices and hour-long games on the weekends (he is a midfielder and runs continuously). He reduces his NPH dose in the morning by 30 percent or more if he has two games in one day. He also reduces his NPH bedtime dose by 50 percent after a day of soccer games or practice. He eats snacks more frequently when he exercises and eats meals with higher amounts of protein. If his practice is at

6:00 P.M., he does not change his morning dose of insulin, but he reduces his dinner Humalog and bedtime NPH doses.

For soccer, a pump user disconnects his pump. He decreases his preexercise meal Humalog bolus a small amount if he is going to play (i.e., 1.7 units versus 2.0 units). He drinks a sport drink during the activity, starting after 10 to 20 minutes, and he tries to begin exercise with a blood sugar of 140 mg/dl or higher.

For recreational soccer, an Ultralente user drinks a sport drink during the activity to maintain her blood sugar levels. Following the activity, she decreases her evening doses of Regular and Ultralente by 2 units each.

Intensity, Duration, and Other Effects

Effect of intensity. For moderate-intensity play, a pump user usually makes no major adjustments to his insulin dose. He eats fruit (oranges or bananas) on the sidelines. In a stressful or intense playing situation, he sometimes decreases his basal rate by 33 percent (from 0.6 to 0.4 units per hour). Occasionally, in wet or slippery situations, he removes his pump. He finds that his blood sugar begins to rise after about an hour off the pump.

Effect of seasonal play. For practices and games, an Ultralente user may reduce her preworkout Humalog insulin by a couple of units. During the season her Ultralente dose is lower both in the morning (from 21 to 14 units) and the evening (from 10 to 7 units).

CROSS-COUNTRY SKIING

Cross-country skiing is one of the best overall aerobic exercises you can do. Athletes who participate regularly in this activity can become very aerobically fit. "Skiing" on the NordicTrack (see chapter 9) can bestow similar benefits, although most people do not do this activity for as long as they would ski outdoors. Your changes in diet and insulin will depend mainly on the duration of the activity and the environmental conditions (i.e., temperature and wind chill).

The duration of cross-country skiing will be the most important factor affecting regimen changes. Longer-duration skiing will result in greater muscle glycogen depletion and increase the risk of later-onset hypoglycemia. You will need greater regimen changes (both reduced insulin and increased carbohydrate intake) for prolonged skiing. Another effect will come from the cold conditions of skiing. Greater carbohydrate usage occurs in colder environments, despite the increased heat production that occurs while you exercise. For colder skiing conditions, you will need to make greater regimen changes.

Athlete Examples

The following real-life examples show that you can make many combinations of regimen changes to compensate for cross-country ski-

CROSS-COUNTRY SKIING

User	Insulin	Diet
NPH/Lente	• For shorter-duration skiing (1 hour or less), reduce short-acting insulin by 10-25% for meals preceding the activity. • For longer durations (2 hours or more), reduce short-acting insulin by 25-50%. • Reduce morning doses of NPH (if taken) by 20-30% as well for more prolonged skiing.	• For shorter durations, supplement with a carbohydrate intake of 15-20 grams per hour. • For longer durations, increase carbohydrate intake by 15-30 grams per hour, depending on insulin reductions.
Insulin Pump	• For skiing an hour or less, reduce basal insulin rates by 50-100% during the activity. Make this change by itself or in combination with a 25-40% reduction in meal boluses before exercise. • For skiing 2 hours or more, both reductions in basal rates and boluses will likely be necessary.	• For shorter skiing, increase carbohydrate intake by 15-20 grams per hour if basal insulin or boluses are not reduced. • For longer durations, additional carbohydrate (15-30 grams per hour) may be necessary depending on insulin reductions.
Ultralente	• For skiing an hour or less, reduce short-acting insulin dose by 10-25% for meals before the activity. • For longer durations (2 hours or more), reduce short-acting insulin by 25-50%, depending on circulating insulin levels during the activity. • Reduce morning Ultralente doses by 20-30% as well for all-day skiing.	• Increases in carbohydrate intake of 15-20 grams may replace the reductions in short-acting insulin for shorter-duration skiing. • Increase carbohydrate by 15-30 grams per hour for longer-duration skiing along with making reductions in insulin doses.

ing, depending on the length of the activity and circulating levels of insulin.

Insulin Changes Alone

For cross-country skiing, an NPH user decreases her short-acting (Regular) insulin by 15 to 20 percent. She finds that her blood sugars tend to drop more following the activity than during it, so she needs to eat more afterward. A pump user decreases her preexercise meal bolus by 50 percent and decreases her basal rate by 50 to 75 percent while exercising. An Ultralente user goes cross-country skiing on the weekends during the winter. She does not change her Ultralente dose, but she decreases her lunch Humalog dose from 6 units to 1 unit while skiing.

Combined Insulin and Diet Changes

For cross-country skiing all day, an NPH user reduces her NPH insulin by 3 to 5 units (from 23 to 20 or 18) and her Regular insulin by 2 units in the morning. In the evening, she cuts back her NPH by 1 to 2 units and her Regular dose by 1 unit. She also eats more food while skiing, especially for breakfast, lunch, and snacks.

Another NPH user has done day trips as well as overnight camping trips of cross-country skiing. She finds that sleeping in a tent, especially in the cold, requires less insulin, so the first night of her trip she reduces her bedtime NPH dose by 30 percent. During the day while skiing with her backpack, she usually reduces all Humalog doses by 20 to 30 percent and increases her carbohydrate intake by 50 percent by snacking during the activity.

A pump user decreases her basal rate by 50 percent during cross-country skiing for one to three hours. She only eats periodically while exercising, but she takes only a third of her usual bolus for meals and snacks while exercising.

An Ultralente user decreases both his Humalog insulin (by 50 percent) and his morning Ultralente dose (by 2 to 3 units down from 15 units) for vigorous, all-day cross-country skiing. He may also add solid or liquid carbohydrates depending on his blood sugar levels during the day.

Intensity, Duration, and Other Effects

Effect of duration. An Ultralente user participates in cross-country ski races of 50 kilometers or more. In training, he averages 20 to 25 kilometers per day. For races, he decreases his Ultralente insulin by 50 percent in the morning (normally 4 units reduced to 2) and eats additional carbohydrates before and during the race. For his regular training, he only adds carbohydrates but does not adjust his insulin dose.

Effect of circulating insulin levels. An NPH user who only takes NPH at bedtime will reduce his short-acting insulin (Regular) by 50 percent for cross-country skiing if he exercises less than four hours after taking it. If the exercise is more than four hours after insulin dosage, he makes no adjustment to his short-acting insulin.

ROWING

This activity is usually aerobic in nature, as it is sustained for longer than two minutes. Crew regattas (races on open water) may actually be more intense and last for a shorter period of time and can have a larger anaerobic component (involving the lactic acid system and other anaerobic sources of energy) than other forms of rowing. Wind conditions can also affect rowing. This activity can be quite intense as it involves full-body musculature and a significant amount of upper-body muscular work. Regimen changes (insulin and diet) will depend on the intensity and duration of the activity.

The intensity and duration of rowing have the biggest effects on blood sugars. Actual open-water crewing events like crew regattas (races) will usually be more intense and shorter in duration, resulting in a larger hormonal response that may raise blood sugar levels as well as a greater use of anaerobic energy (lactic acid system). During these events, blood sugars will be easier to maintain and may actually rise following short events. Longer, less intense rowing (during practices) may require greater regimen changes to maintain blood sugar levels. Wind conditions can also increase the intensity of rowing (stronger winds will provide a greater resistance).

Athlete Examples

These real-life examples show that exercise timing and starting blood sugar levels affect the need for regimen changes.

ROWING

User	Insulin	Diet
NPH/Lente	• Reduce doses of short-acting insulins by 10-20% before short, intense bouts of rowing. • Reduce doses of morning NPH or Lente (if taken) by 10-20% for afternoon exercise. • Make minimal changes in short-acting insulin doses for activity 3-4 hours after an injection, especially if only short-acting insulins are used during the day. • For longer-duration, less-intense rowing (30 minutes or more), reduce insulin by 20-30%, depending on the duration of rowing and carbohydrate intake.	• Shorter rowing bouts may require 10-20 grams of extra carbohydrate, depending on the reductions in insulin and exercise duration. • Carbohydrate supplementation up to 30 grams or more may be needed for longer duration rowing.
Insulin Pump	• For shorter, more intense rowing, reduce basal insulin rates during the activity by 25-50%. • Complete removal or suspension of the pump may actually result in increased blood sugar levels due to the glucose-raising hormones released during more intense exercise. If this occurs, give a small bolus of insulin when reconnecting. • Small reductions in meal boluses (10-20%) before the activity may be necessary. • For longer, less intense rowing lasting 30 minutes or more, reductions of 25-100% in basal rates and 20-30% reductions in insulin boluses may be needed.	• Supplement with 15-30 grams of carbohydrate per hour, depending on reductions in insulin and duration of rowing. • With any reductions in insulin, minimal carbohydrate supplementation may be necessary for intense rowing bouts.
Ultralente	• Reduce short-acting insulin doses by 10-20% before shorter, more intense bouts of rowing. • For longer, less intense rowing of 30 minutes or more, reduce short-acting insulin by 20-30%, depending on the planned duration of rowing.	• Depending on the duration of rowing and reductions in insulin, supplement with up to 15-30 grams of carbohydrate. • For intense exercise 3-4 hours following the last injection, minimal supplementation (0-15 grams) may be required even without reducing the last insulin dose. • Usually no changes in Ultralente doses are necessary.

Intensity, Duration, and Other Effects

Effect of time of day. An NPH user rows twice weekly on open water. For this activity, which he does before breakfast and his morning insulin dose of Regular and NPH, he does not make any insulin adjustments because he takes his insulin after his exercise. If his fasting blood sugar is 60 to 70 mg/dl, he eats a piece of fruit before exercising.

Effect of fasting blood sugars. A Lente user sculls for two to three hours on weekends without changing his Lente dose. He rows early in the morning, so he skips his morning dose of Regular and Humalog, eats his usual breakfast just before beginning the exercise, and carries Humalog with him in case he needs a small amount later in the exercise. He has found that his starting blood sugar affects his need to eat extra food. If his blood sugar is near 200 mg/dl, he will not eat anything. If it is more than 200, he takes 1 to 3 units of Humalog before exercising. A starting blood sugar of much less than 140 mg/dl impairs his workout.

SWIMMING

This activity is mainly aerobic in nature, especially when swimming longer distances rather than competing in short races. Longer-endurance swims are aerobic in nature, utilizing a mixture fats and carbohydrates. Carbohydrate use (blood sugar and muscle glycogen) increases with greater-intensity swimming. Shorter sprints or racing competitions (covering distances of 200 yards or less) may utilize mainly anaerobic systems (phosphagens and lactic acid systems). You can make alterations in insulin, food intake, or both, depending on the intensity and duration of the activity, the time of day you swim, and starting blood sugar levels.

Swimming intensity, duration, timing, and starting blood sugar levels have the biggest effects on blood sugar control for all regimens. Swimming intensity will affect the release of glucose-raising hormones: more intense exercise such as swim meets or other competitions involving short, intense swimming results in a possible increase in blood sugar levels rather than a decrease. Longer swims will result in a greater use of muscle and liver glycogen, thus increasing insulin sensitivity following the exercise and the risk for later-onset hypoglycemia. Circulating insulin levels will also affect your need for carbohydrate supplementation. If you swim when

SWIMMING

User	Insulin	Diet
NPH/Lente	• Short swimming sprints (like at swim meets) will usually require minimal alterations in insulin or food. • For more prolonged, continuous endurance swimming of 30 minutes or more, reduce short-acting insulins by 25-50%, depending on swim duration and carbohydrate intake. • Reduce morning doses of NPH or Lente (if taken) by 10-30% for afternoon swims. • Reduce short-acting insulin doses by 10-30% for meals following the swim if it was prolonged. • Consider reducing bedtime doses of NPH or Lente by 10-20%, especially following more prolonged swims.	• Consume an extra 15-30 grams of carbohydrate per hour for longer swims, depending on the reductions in insulin. • Eat an extra bedtime snack to prevent overnight hypoglycemia following longer swimming workouts. • When swims are done when circulating insulin levels are lower (in the early morning or 3-4 hours after the last injection of short-acting insulin), make smaller increases in food.
Insulin Pump	• If you remove your pump during swimming (which provides the most normal insulin response to exercise), you will need little or no carbohydrate supplementation except maybe for prolonged swims (over an hour). • Short, intense swims (like at meets) may actually cause blood sugar levels to rise. Give a small bolus of insulin should hyperglycemia occur. • If you wear a waterproof pump during swims, reduce basal rates by 25-75% during the activity, depending on intensity and duration of the activity. • Reduce meal boluses (within 3-4 hours before the activity) by 10-30% to minimize circulating insulin levels during the swim. • Reduce bolus by 10-25% for meals afterward, especially following longer workouts. • Keep the basal rate lowered by 10-20% for several hours after the swim to prevent hypoglycemia after long or unusual swims.	• The amount of carbohydrate you need depends on the length of the swim, time of day you swim, starting blood sugar levels, and reductions in insulin. • Eat 15-30 grams of carbohydrate per hour for most swims. • Consume 0-15 grams of carbohydrate for early-morning swims due to increased insulin resistance at that time of day. • Eat extra snacks (especially at bedtime) following prolonged swims to prevent later-onset hypoglycemia.

(continued)

SWIMMING *(continued)*

User	Insulin	Diet
Ultralente	• Make minimal alterations in insulin or carbohydrate intake for short swimming sprints. • Reduce short-acting insulin doses by 10-30% for longer swims (if within 3-4 hours of the last insulin taken), depending on the length of the swim. • Reduce insulin doses by 10-25% for meals after the swim, especially following more prolonged swims. • Consider reducing evening Ultralente doses by 10-20% following unusually long workouts or multiple days of swimming.	• Increase carbohydrates by 15-30 grams per hour for longer swims, depending on reductions in short-acting insulin. • Consume fewer carbohydrate (0-20 grams) for swims early in the morning (when insulin resistance is high), or more than 3-4 hours after the last injection of short-acting insulin, or for more intense swimming. • For shorter or more intense swims, make minimal increases in carbohydrate (0-20 grams) as well. • Eat extra snacks following the activity (especially at bedtime) to prevent later-onset hypoglycemia.

levels of short-acting insulins are minimal (more than three to four hours after the last short-acting insulin dose or with lowered basal rates for pump users), blood sugars will not decrease as much; the body's glycemic response is more normal due to lower insulin levels. Even if you exercise during times of lower circulating insulin, you may need to supplement with extra carbohydrate during prolonged swims (more than one hour) due to the depletion of muscle and liver glycogen stores. If you swim before breakfast you will have more stable blood sugar levels with less of a need for extra carbohydrate. If your blood sugars are higher in the morning, you may actually need a small dose of short-acting insulin to prevent a rise in blood sugars by the end of the swim. Higher blood sugars at a later time of day may require less of an adjustment as swimming will usually cause them to drop.

Athlete Examples

The following swimming examples show that the duration and intensity of swimming as well as the time of day you exercise largely determine the best regimen changes.

Insulin Changes Alone

For swimming 20 minutes after lunch, an NPH user usually decreases her prelunch Humalog by 15 percent and her bedtime NPH by 15 percent. She finds that if she does not swim for two days in a row, she needs to increase her lunch Humalog by 30 percent and her bedtime NPH by 20 percent.

Diet Changes Alone

For swimming or water polo, an NPH user eats at least 15 grams of carbohydrate before beginning either activity, depending on her blood glucose levels, but without making any insulin adjustments.

For swimming in the ocean, another NPH user makes sure that his blood sugar is not dropping and that it is somewhat elevated (150 to 200 mg/dl) when he goes out for 30 minutes. He supplements with additional carbohydrates before and after the activity as needed.

For swimming in the morning before his insulin dose, an Ultralente user does not make any insulin adjustments. He drinks a regular soda so that his blood sugar is 225 mg/dl at the beginning and 80 at the end of his one-mile swim.

Combined Insulin and Diet Changes

An NPH user trains regularly with a Masters swim team. For their one-hour workouts, she maintains her usual food intake, but she reduces her Regular preexercise insulin by 1 to 2 units. She eats extra food before swimming for blood sugars below 180 mg/dl.

For an hour of moderate swimming (2,500 yards), a pump user disconnects her pump. In doing so, she finds that she does not normally need any additional carbohydrate to maintain her blood sugar. If she has taken a large bolus for meals within 1 to 2 hours before swimming (4 units of Humalog or more), then her blood sugar will drop during the swim if she does not eat 15 to 20 additional grams of carbohydrates before swimming. She reduces her bolus by about 25 percent for food that she eats soon after swimming.

Intensity, Duration, and Other Effects

Effect of intensity. An NPH user participates in swim team practices lasting 1.5 hours. He finds that a workout decreases his blood glucose level by 130 mg/dl; consequently, his blood sugar level needs to be 200 mg/dl at the start of his workout. He eats carbohydrates to raise his blood sugar (15 grams of carbohydrate raises his blood sugar 60 mg/dl) before swimming, but he does not adjust his insulin doses. Swim meets cause his blood sugars to rise, though, and he needs to take Humalog with any food he eats during meets.

Effect of training volume. An NPH user participates in competitive, year-round swim training that includes four hours of swimming a day (14,000 to 18,000 yards) in two workouts. His training is so consistent that he makes few insulin adjustments on a daily basis. When his training starts to taper for a meet, though, he increases his morning dose of NPH by 2 units and takes a lunch dose of Humalog (6 units plus extra for correction of elevated blood sugars) and may reduce his intake of snacks.

During the swim team season, an Ultralente user reduces her Ultralente dose both in the morning (from 21 to 14 units) and the evening (from 10 to 7 units).

CYCLING

This activity is generally very aerobic in nature. Some cycling events can involve sprinting and intermittent increases in intensity (e.g., hill climbing), both of which will provide a greater stress to anaerobic energy systems, especially the lactic acid system. Carbohydrate use (including both blood glucose and muscle glycogen use) increases with more intense cycling. Road cycling tends to be more prolonged and more intense than stationary cycling and will consequently require more regimen adjustments to compensate. With any insulin regimen, the choices are to lower insulin doses, increase food intake, or both, depending on other factors such as the time of day you exercise, your blood sugar levels, and intensity and duration of the activity.

Cycling intensity and duration, timing of exercise, and starting blood sugar levels will affect blood sugar responses. It will be harder to maintain blood sugar levels during longer-duration cycling (two or more hours) without a combination of carbohydrate supplementation and insulin reductions. Longer rides will also result in greater use of muscle glycogen stores, thus increasing the risk for hypoglycemia following exercise. If you cycle when circulating insulin levels

CYCLING

User	Insulin	Diet
NPH/Lente	• For shorter cycling durations (less than 1 hour) following a meal, reduce short-acting insulin doses by 10-30%. • For planned afternoon cycling, reduce morning doses of NPH or Lente (if taken) by 10-30%. • For longer-duration cycling lasting 1-4 hours or more, reduce insulin by 30-50%. • Reduce short-acting insulin doses by 10-30% for the meal following cycling depending on the duration of the activity. • After longer cycling bouts, consider reducing bedtime doses of NPH or Lente by 10-20% as well to prevent nocturnal hypoglycemia.	• Supplement with up to 15 grams of carbohydrate for shorter-duration cycling. • Less food may be necessary for exercise when circulating insulin levels are lower, such as 3-4 hours following a meal, especially if NPH or Lente doses are at bedtime only. • For longer-duration cycling, consume 15-30 grams of carbohydrate per hour depending on the insulin reductions. • For cycling in the morning before breakfast, supplement with minimal carbohydrate for shorter distances, and only after the first 30-45 minutes of the activity. • Possibly eat additional food following the activity to prevent low blood sugars. • A bedtime snack may be necessary if evening insulin doses are not reduced following prolonged cycling bouts.
Insulin Pump	• For shorter cycling distances, reduce basal rates by 25-50%, or suspend basal rates altogether to achieve a more normal physiological response to exercise. • Supplement with less carbohydrate for cycling in the morning before breakfast due to higher insulin resistance at that time of day. • For longer cycling (1-4 hours or more), reduce boluses by 30-50% for meals preceding exercise as well as for meals immediately following the activity, depending on the extra carbohydrates consumed during cycling and basal rate reductions. • Consider reducing basal rates 30-60 minutes before beginning exercise and maintain the lower basal level for several hours or even overnight following longer cycling distances to prevent later-onset hypoglycemia.	• Consume up to 15-30 grams of additional carbohydrate for every 30-60 minutes of cycling, depending on exercise intensity. • Consume extra carbohydrate following prolonged cycling to prevent post-exercise hypoglycemia. • Consider eating an extra bedtime snack if basal rates are not lowered overnight following prolonged bouts of cycling.

(continued)

CYCLING *(continued)*

User	Insulin	Diet
Ultralente	• Minimize circulating insulin levels during cycling by exercising 3-4 hours after last injection of short-acting insulin (2-3 hours after a Humalog injection). • If exercise begins fairly soon after a meal, reduce short-acting insulin doses by 10-30% for shorter or more intense cycling. • For longer-duration cycling, reduce preexercise meal short-acting insulin doses by 30-50%. • Reduce insulin doses for meals following the activity by 10-30% to prevent hypoglycemia later in the day. • For exceptionally long cycling bouts, consider reducing evening Ultralente doses by 10-20%.	• Consume 15-30 grams of carbohydrate per 30-60 minutes of cycling, depending on insulin reductions, especially if cycling after a meal. • You will need minimal carbohydrate supplementation for shorter cycling distances, especially if exercise is done more than 3-4 hours after the last dose of short-acting insulin. • Consume extra carbohydrate following prolonged cycling to prevent post-exercise hypoglycemia. • Consider eating an extra bedtime snack if you do not lower your basal rates overnight following prolonged bouts of cycling.

are lower, either in the morning or before meals (when you take only short-acting insulins), then cycling will not cause blood sugar levels to drop as much because circulating insulin levels will be lower and more "normal." If blood sugars are high in the morning (more than 200 mg/dl), you may need a small dose of short-acting insulin before exercise to prevent a rise in blood sugars while cycling. Higher blood sugars later in the day will probably respond better to the exercise, and your blood sugars will decrease more.

Athlete Examples

Athletes decrease their insulin and increase their food intake to compensate for cycling, depending on their starting blood sugars and circulating insulin levels. More prolonged cycling bouts require greater regimen changes.

Insulin Changes Alone

An NPH user bikes 15 to 30 miles daily. For cycling after lunch, he reduces his prelunch Humalog from 5.5 units to 1 unit for his normal food intake. When he participates in multiple-day biking events, he also decreases his bedtime dose of NPH slightly.

Diet Changes Alone

For recreational cycling for one to two hours, another NPH user avoids exercising immediately after a meal when his Humalog dose is at its peak. Instead, he prefers to cycle immediately before a meal when Humalog levels are low. He eats two to three fruits before biking and uses rapid carbohydrate snacks (sport drinks, PowerBars, and gels) during the ride. He tries to take two-thirds of the carbohydrates during the exercise and one-third following exercise, especially pasta at the next meal, because he rarely gets low blood sugars during the exercise but he often gets low blood sugars afterward.

For cycling 30 kilometers or more at a time in the late afternoon, another pump user first tests his blood sugar several times to establish a trend. Starting with his blood sugar in a normal range, he supplements with fruit, Fig Newtons, and squirts of juice or water from a bottle every 5 to 10 minutes during his ride. He maintains his basal rate and makes no real adjustments to his insulin dose for this activity.

An Ultralente user cycles 30 minutes to two hours on weekdays. For this activity, she eats additional carbohydrate but does not change her insulin because she cycles before meals when she experiences minimal effects from her last Humalog injection.

Combined Insulin and Diet Changes

For short rides of 10 miles or less, an NPH user eats an additional 10 grams of carbohydrate. For longer day rides, she reduces her Humalog doses by 20 percent and eats extra carbohydrate. For a one-month bike trip in Australia, she needed to cut all her insulin doses by 60 percent or more and increase her carbohydrate intake by 50 to 75 percent.

For cycling an hour, a Lente user eats 125 to 150 calories worth of carbohydrates (including one-half of a banana and one-fourth of bagel) and hydrates well before the exercise. His starting blood sugar determines how much he needs to eat for the activity: if his blood sugar is near 200 mg/dl, he will not eat anything; if it is more than 200, he takes 1 to 3 units of Humalog before exercising, according to his blood sugar level. Starting with a blood sugar much less than 140 mg/dl impairs his workout. He also tries to separate his short-acting insulin shots and any activity by three hours or more. He does not change his Lente dose at all.

An insulin pump user cycles for 90 minutes on weekdays and for four to five hours on weekends. For these activities, she reduces her normal basal amount by one-third (typically from 0.3 units per hour to 0.2 units). She also eats (without bolusing) a PowerBar every 45 minutes and supplements with a sport drink as needed every 30 minutes. Immediately after a long workout (four to five hours), if her blood sugar levels are normal, she has to take a 2-unit bolus to keep her blood sugar levels from rising. Later on she experiences postexercise late-onset hypoglycemia and has to reduce her basal rates by 20 percent or more during the night.

Another pump user cycles intensely for two to five hours on a daily basis. To manage this level of activity, he decreases his preexercise meal bolus by 20 to 50 percent (depending on the length of the ride) if he is going to begin within 60 to 90 minutes after eating. He reduces his basal rate by 50 to 60 percent one hour before he begins exercising and returns it to normal 30 minutes before completion of exercise, especially if he plans on eating immediately afterward. While riding he drinks a sport drink every two hours (35 to 40 grams) and eats 18 grams of a PowerBar.

For cycling 45 minutes to two hours, an Ultralente user always eats extra carbohydrates (fruit, Coke, granola bars, sport drinks) and reduces his preexercise meal regular dose by 50 to 60 percent. If he cycles for five hours, he also decreases his Ultralente dose in the morning by about 50 percent (from 12 units to 5 or 6 units), and then he may increase his evening dose by 2 units or so (from 5 up to 7 units) to compensate for the large decrease in the morning.

Another Ultralente user participates in intense cycle training and racing. He rides for two to four hours a day for a total of 200 to 250 miles a week. On longer rides, he eats half a PowerBar every 30 to 45 minutes. He also takes 5 units of regular insulin after exercising and eats a large amount of carbohydrate to replenish his muscle glycogen stores. He may increase his bedtime snack depending on the intensity and duration of his ride that day. He may lower his bedtime-only Ultralente dose by 1 to 2 units.

Intensity, Duration, and Other Effects

Effect of intensity and duration. For intense or longer workouts (60 miles or more), an NPH user decreases his Regular insulin by 1 to 2 units in the preceding meal. For an hour or less of cycling at an easy pace, he does not reduce his insulin and needs to supplement very little with extra carbohydrate. For long cycling trips (100 miles), an insulin pump user has to suspend her pump altogether and eat frequently without bolusing any insulin for the food to prevent hypoglycemia.

Effect of multiple days of cycling. An NPH user varies his regimen based on his previous days of exercise. On the first day of cycling 30 to 45 minutes in the morning (after one or more days of not working out), he makes no immediate adjustments to his morning insulin (usually 2 units of Humalog and 10 units of NPH), but he may cut his Humalog by 1 unit at dinner and his NPH by 1 unit at bedtime. On the second day, he additionally reduces his morning dose by 1 unit each. On the third day, he reduces his morning doses by 2 units each and also reduces his dinner and bedtime doses by 1 to 2 units. He also may increase his carbohydrate intake during the day and his bedtime snack.

TRIATHLONS

These activities include mini (sprint), half, and full-length triathlon events. By nature, they are all prolonged activities that almost exclusively utilize aerobic energy systems. Half and full-length events stress endurance and cause significant glycogen depletion from muscles. The body mainly uses fat and carbohydrate for any of these events, and carbohydrate use (both blood glucose and muscle glycogen) increases with exercise intensity. Actual responses will vary with the duration and intensity of the event. You can make alterations in insulin, diet, or both, but for the longer triathlons, alterations in insulin may be absolutely necessary to avoid hypoglycemia during and after the event.

The length of the triathlon will greatly affect the response to the exercise. Minitriathlons may be completed with an hour of intensive exercise. Half and full-length events can last three to eight hours and cause significant glycogen depletion in most active muscles. Carbohydrate use can be significant during both greater-intensity, shorter-duration events and less intense, longer-duration events. However, with the longer events, alterations in insulin may be absolutely necessary to avoid hypoglycemia during and after the event compared with shorter events that result in a greater release of glucose-raising hormones as well as a reduced glycogen depletion.

Athlete Examples

These examples show the varieties of regimen changes determined largely by the length of the event. Longer triathlons require major insulin and food intake changes for maintenance of blood sugars.

Combined Insulin and Diet Changes

For triathlons at the international level, an NPH user varies her regimen according to her starting blood sugar levels. For events lasting more than two hours, she does not make any adjustments to her insulin if her starting blood sugar levels are more than 180 mg/dl, but she supplements 15 grams of carbohydrate every 45 minutes. If she starts at less than 108 mg/dl, she decreases her Humalog dose by 2 units before and after the exercise, and she supplements 20 to 30 grams of carbohydrate every 40 minutes. She tests her blood sugar more often during long events so that she can determine whether her blood sugar levels are going up or down.

An insulin pump user participates in triathlons and training, including the Hawaii Ironman. For these activities, she reduces her normal basal amount by a third (typically from 0.3 units per hour to 0.2 units). She also eats (without bolusing) a PowerBar every 45 minutes and supplements with a sport drink as needed every 30 minutes or so and drinks water as well. During the swimming portion, she disconnects her pump most of the time. She finds that immediately after a long training workout (four to five hours), if her blood sugar levels are normal, she has to take a 2-unit bolus to keep her blood sugar levels from rising. Later she tends to experience postexercise late-onset hypoglycemia and has to reduce her basal rates during the night.

For triathlons, an Ultralente user decreases his morning short-acting insulin by taking 3 to 4 units of Regular only with no

TRIATHLONS

User	Insulin	Diet
NPH/Lente	• Insulin changes will vary widely with the length of the triathlon event. • Reduce pre-event evening NPH or Lente dose by up to 50%, but realize that doing so will result in higher blood sugar levels in the morning before the event. • Short events will require a 25-50% reduction in short-acting insulin before the exercise. • Reduce both morning NPH or Lente (if taken) and the shorter-acting insulin before longer events by 25-75% each, depending on fasting blood sugar levels. • Postevent meals may require a 20-30% reduction of short-acting insulin (or more for prolonged events) while insulin sensitivity remains heightened. • Reduce the evening NPH or Lente dose by 10-30%, and eat an additional bedtime snack to prevent nocturnal hypoglycemia, especially if the triathlon was a prolonged event resulting in significant depletion of muscle glycogen.	• For sprint triathlons, eat an additional 15-30 grams of carbohydrate, depending on starting blood sugar levels. • For longer events, supplement with 15-30 grams of carbohydrate for every 30-45 minutes of exercise, depending on blood sugar levels and insulin reductions. • Starting with a higher blood sugar will usually require less carbohydrate supplementation during the event, at least during the first hour of exercise.
Insulin Pump	• Do not alter basal insulin rates or boluses until the morning of the competition. • Reduce the basal rate during the triathlon by 25-100% depending on the length of the event. • The basal rate can be reduced starting 1-2 hours before exercise to minimize circulating insulin levels, if desired. • For sprint triathlons, it is most effective to suspend or remove the pump altogether. • Reduce meal insulin boluses preceding the event by 25-75% depending on fasting blood sugar levels, expected basal rate reductions, and the length of the triathlon.	• Supplement with 15-30 grams of carbohydrate for every 30-45 minutes of exercise during the event, especially a longer event, depending on blood sugar levels and insulin reductions. • Sprint triathlons may not require any food intake during the event if basal insulin levels have been sufficiently lowered. • Longer events may also necessitate eating extra food following the event (with minimal insulin coverage) as well as an additional bedtime snack.

(continued)

TRIATHLONS *(continued)*

User	Insulin	Diet
Insulin Pump	• During the swimming portion, disconnect the pump, or reduce the basal rate to a minimal amount (waterproof pumps only). • Take fewer insulin boluses (20-30%) for food eaten after the event and even more following prolonged events. • Consider reducing basal insulin rates by 10-25% during the rest of the day and overnight to lower the risk of postexercise late-onset hypoglycemia.	
Ultralente	• Reduce morning short-acting insulin dose before the event by 25-75%, depending on fasting blood sugar levels. • Reduce the morning Ultralente dose by 10-50% depending on the duration of the event. • Reduce Ultralente less for shorter events than for longer events. • Consider reducing the evening dose of Ultralente, as well, but to a lesser extent than in the morning (10-20%), especially if the reduction in the morning dose was large. • Reduce doses of short-acting insulin following the event by at least 20-30%. The more significant the muscle glycogen depletion is, the greater the reduction you need.	• You may not need any food intake during shorter events (sprint triathlons) if circulating insulin levels are low. • For longer events, supplement with 15-30 grams of carbohydrate for every 30-45 minutes of exercise depending on blood sugar levels and insulin reductions. • Longer events may also warrant extra food intake following the event and a bedtime snack to prevent later-onset hypoglycemia.

Humalog (usually he takes 4 units of each). He tries to begin a race with his blood sugar between 150 and 200 mg/dl, and then he supplements with PowerBars during the event, taking a half of a bar every 30 minutes. After exercise he tends to use Regular insulin instead of Humalog because it gets into his system a lot more slowly. He does not adjust his Ultralente dose.

For full Ironman triathlons, another Ultralente user decreases his morning dose of Regular insulin by 50 to 60 percent and supplements with carbohydrates (fruit, regular soda, granola bars, or carbohydrate drinks). He may also decrease his Ultralente dose in the morning by up to 50 percent (from 12 units to 5 or 6 units), and then he may increase his evening dose by 2 units or so (from 5 up to 7 units) to compensate for the large decrease in the morning.

Intensity, Duration, and Other Effects

Effect of seasonal training. In the off-season when one NPH user only exercises 15 hours a week on average, she has to take 3 to 4 units more for slightly smaller meals as she is not doing back-to-back long, hard exercise sessions. During the season she trains 25 to 30 hours a week at varying intensities (one to three sessions a day) and finds that she needs 2 to 4 units less insulin for every meal while eating more daily carbohydrates and during her two-hour exercise sessions. She tests her blood sugar levels before, during, and after all exercise sessions.

ULTRAENDURANCE EVENTS AND TRAINING

These types of activities include multiple days of strenuous exercise (cycling, running, walking, backpacking) as well as ultramarathons and other extremely prolonged distance events. Prolonged events almost exclusively utilize aerobic energy systems. Fuel utilization is a mix of muscle glycogen and blood glucose, circulating and intramuscular lipids (fats), and even protein sources. Training for and competing in ultraendurance events can maximally stress the body's stores of energy, resulting in a significant depletion. You will need changes in insulin and diet during the event as well as for 24 to 48 hours following the event during the repletion of various energy sources in the body. Insulin sensitivity will generally be heightened during this time, and the risk for hypoglycemia is greater, especially without appropriate compensation.

The length of the exercise will greatly affect the blood sugar response. Events or training lasting three to eight hours will cause significant glycogen depletion from most active muscles. Carbohydrate use (both blood glucose and muscle glycogen) can be significant during these longer-duration events and training. With longer exercise participation, you will definitely need alterations in insulin to avoid hypoglycemia during the event and afterward due to the extreme level of muscle glycogen depletion.

Athlete Examples

These examples show the extreme regimen changes that are necessary for ultraendurance events and training. The type and length of the event or training determine the changes, and changes always include both insulin and food intake adjustments.

Combined Insulin and Diet Changes

An NPH user participates in triathlons at the international level. For events lasting more than two hours, she does not make any adjustments to her insulin if her starting blood sugar levels are more than 180 mg/dl. At that level, she supplements with 15 grams of carbohydrate every 45 minutes. If she starts at less than 108 mg/dl, she decreases her Humalog dose by 2 units before and after the exercise, and she supplements with 20 to 30 grams of carbohydrate every 40 minutes. She tests her blood sugar more often during long events so that she can determine whether her blood sugar levels are going up or down. For the off-season when she is not doing back-to-back workouts, she generally has to take 3 to 4 more units of short-acting insulin for slightly smaller meals.

A pump user participates in Double Century cycling races (200 miles) and full-length triathlons and reduces her normal basal insulin by a third (typically from 0.3 units per hour to 0.2 units). She also eats (without bolusing) a PowerBar every 45 minutes and supplements with a sport drink as needed every 30 minutes or so and drinks water. She finds that immediately after a long workout, if her blood sugar levels are normal, she has to take a 2-unit bolus to keep her blood sugar from rising. Later she tends to experience postexercise late-onset hypoglycemia and has to reduce her basal rates during the night.

Another pump user is a racewalker who usually walks 25 miles a day. He has participated in walks across the United States over three summers. For this extended activity, he cuts his basal rate by almost 50 percent. He keeps his Humalog boluses the same, but he eats more food. It works well for him to eat a slow-acting energy bar twice a day while walking all day. He also ingests 10 to 20 grams of carbohydrate every hour and tests his blood sugar frequently.

ULTRAENDURANCE EVENTS AND TRAINING*

User	Insulin	Diet
NPH/Lente	• Reduce your NPH or Lente dose for the previous evening by up to 50% if desired, but expect that doing so will result in higher blood sugar levels in the morning before exercise. • Reduce both the premeal NPH or Lente (if taken) and short-acting insulins before the event by 25-75% each, depending on the fasting blood sugar levels and expected duration of the activity. • Reduce evening NPH or Lente doses following participation by 10-40% to prevent nocturnal hypoglycemia, especially following prolonged events or training that result in significant depletion of muscle glycogen stores.	• Supplement with 15-45 grams of carbohydrate for every 30-45 minutes of exercise, depending on blood sugar levels and reductions in insulin. • Starting with a higher blood sugar will usually require less supplementation during the activity, at least during the first hour. • Postexercise meals usually require a 25-50% reduction of short-acting insulin while insulin sensitivity remains heightened. • Consider eating an additional bedtime snack.
Insulin Pump	• Do not alter basal insulin rates until the morning of the event or training. • Reduce the basal rate during the activity by 25-100% depending on the length of exercise. • Lower your basal insulin rate starting 1-2 hours before exercise begins to minimize circulating insulin levels, if desired. • Reduce preexercise meal boluses by 25-75%, depending on starting blood sugar levels and the expected duration of the activity. • Reduce boluses by 25-50% for meals later in the day depending on blood sugar readings and the amount of exercise done. • Reduce basal insulin rates by at least 10-25% during the rest of the day and overnight to lower the risk of developing postexercise late-onset hypoglycemia.	• During the activity, supplement with 15-45 grams of carbohydrate for every 30-45 minutes of exercise depending on blood sugar levels and reductions in insulin. • Consume extra food after the event (albeit with lower insulin boluses) and a bedtime snack.
Ultralente	• Reduce morning short-acting insulin dose before the event by 25-75%, depending on fasting blood sugar levels and the expected duration of the activity.	• Supplement with 15-45 grams of carbohydrate for every 30-45 minutes of exercise, depending on blood sugar levels and reductions in insulin.

(continued)

ULTRAENDURANCE EVENTS AND TRAINING *(continued)*

User	Insulin	Diet
Ultralente	• Reduce the morning Ultralente dose by 0-50% depending on the expected duration of the activity. • Reduce doses of short-acting insulin for any food eaten following the event by 25-50%. • Consider reducing the evening dose of Ultralente to a lesser extent (10-20%) but probably not by as much if the reduction in the morning dose was large.	• Eat extra carbohydrate following the event (with reduced insulin amounts) and an additional bedtime snack to prevent later-onset and overnight hypoglycemia.

* Ultraendurance events and training will require combined changes in insulin and diet during the activities as well as for 24-48 hours following participation during the repletion of various energy sources in the body.

An Ultralente user runs 30 to 100 miles at a time, so he reduces his morning dose of Ultralente by 1 unit (from 2 units to 1). If running tough trail races of 100 miles, he takes 0.5 to 0.75 units of Ultralente every 12 hours. While running, he drinks Coke, sport drinks, and water equally. Before races of any length, he eats a normal breakfast (cereal, toast, and milk) but only takes a small amount of Humalog (0 to 1 units instead of his usual 5). He also eats pretzels during 50-kilometer races. For longer races, he eats additional salted cantaloupe, bananas, jelly beans, watermelon, and salty soup (for trail runs).

Another Ultralente user participates in Double Century biking events (200 miles of biking per day, or more than 12 hours). For this event, she takes her usual morning dose of Ultralente and Humalog, reduces her prelunch Humalog by 5 units (from 6 to 1), and reduces her predinner Ultralente by 1 unit and Humalog by 3 units (to 0). Her total food intake during the event is significantly more than usual. For week-long tours of 50 to 100 miles per day (four to seven hours), she keeps her morning dose of Ultralente and Humalog the same initially and decreases her lunch Humalog by 5 units. Her calorie intake increases from about 2,000 calories per day to 3,000 to 3,500 on touring days. Within about 36 to 48 hours of beginning the tour, she starts to decrease her Ultralente dose slightly (by 0.25 to 0.5 unit for both Ultralente doses) and may also decrease her morning Humalog by 0.5 to 1 unit (from 3 units). She keeps her Ultralente dose down for the remainder of the tour and for a few days afterward.

One Ultralente user participated in a Bridge-to-Bridge cycling century, which included climbing 10,000 vertical feet in the North Carolina Blue Ridge Mountains. On the day of the race, he decreased his normal Ultralente dose from 15 units to 10. He kept his breakfast Humalog dose (15 units) and food the same for the event starting 90 minutes after breakfast. On the seven-hour ride, he ate eight bananas, half a bag of chocolate chip cookies, one bunch of grapes, and six granola bars and drank water and a diluted sport drink, all without taking any supplemental Humalog. For dinner he reduced his normal insulin from 17/7 (Ultralente/Humalog) to 12/4, set his alarm for 1:00 A.M., and drank a glass of orange juice in the middle of the night. The next day he returned his Ultralente doses to normal.

Another Ultralente user participated in a 36-hour, no-sleep adventure race in Canada that involved grueling physical activities: 10 hours of strenuous hiking through natural terrain, four hours of canoeing, 10 hours of biking on overgrown, hilly logging roads, more hiking, more biking, and then several hours of white-water rafting, all done continuously. During this event, he took absolutely no short-acting insulin although he ate throughout the race, and he reduced each of his twice-daily Ultralente doses by 25 percent for each injection.

As you can see, many individuals with diabetes safely and successfully participate in all levels of endurance activities, even the extreme ones. With a little practice and a lot of blood sugar checking, even the more moderate exerciser can learn to manage his or her diabetes while participating in frequent endurance exercise.

Chapter 8

Power Sports

We have all heard of Michael Jordan, John Elway, and Mark McGwire because of the popularity of power sports. But have you heard of Chris Dudley, Bobby Clarke, Jason Johnson, Wade Wilson, Jonathan Hayes, Jay Leeuwenberg, and Gary Mabbutt? While they may not be as well known, they are all professional athletes with diabetes playing football, basketball, ice hockey, baseball, and soccer. All people, with or without diabetes, can safely do power sports and other activities. Young adult and youth participation in team sports is the way to go these days! Kids can start early developing their coordination and skill by doing various activities, and adults can stay youthful and active by participating. Check around your area for a local gym, recreation center, or sports league, and get the whole family involved in the activities! The following activities are profiled in this chapter: basketball, volleyball, baseball and softball, field hockey, lacrosse, football and rugby, gymnastics, track and field, ice hockey, water polo, powerlifting, and wrestling. (Look for the ever-popular soccer in chapter 7 as it is considered more of an endurance activity.)

In general, power sports require short, powerful bouts of activity. In baseball, this may involve hitting the ball and sprinting to first base; in basketball, it may be a jump and a dunk of the ball; in track and field, it may be a high jump. These intense activities may have no effect on blood sugars or may actually raise them. In other cases, the activity is so minimal that it has little overall effect on blood sugar levels. When you do intense activities intermittently over a prolonged period of time, the activities have a cumulative effect on glycogen use and may require greater regimen changes in order to prevent blood sugar levels from decreasing. For a fuller explanation of the various energy systems and energy sources used for different types of exercise, refer to chapter 2.

This chapter gives general recommendations for power sports as a whole. Within an individual activity, both general recommendations as well as real-life examples of some people's specific changes in insulin and diet are listed according to insulin regimen (NPH and Lente, pump, and Ultralente users). *Users of oral hypoglycemic agents are not listed separately, but the general recommendations under diet changes alone (or more specifically, diet changes for NPH and Lente users) apply as an approximate guide for people with type 2 diabetes with starting blood sugars in a normal range.* However, when blood sugars are elevated, dietary intake will need to decrease. You should make short-term or long-term reductions in oral doses under the advice of a physician only. For more information about the actions of various types of insulins and oral hypoglycemic agents, refer to chapter 3.

GENERAL RECOMMENDATIONS

Most power sports require "power" performances in the form of short, intense bouts of muscular activity. If the activity lasts less than 10 seconds, the phosphagen system alone provides the required muscular energy. Children are particularly suited for these types of short-burst activities; their other two energy systems are less well developed until they reach adolescence. For power sports, the phosphagen system combines with the lactic acid system to provide the muscular energy for anaerobic activities that last up to two minutes. ATP and creatine phosphate supply the immediate energy, while muscle glycogen mainly supplies the remainder. The sport itself determines the necessary changes in insulin or diet because intense activities can decrease, increase, or have no impact on blood sugar levels. When you do an intensive activity intermittently over an extended period, as with basketball, it can have a cumulative effect on glycogen use and you may need greater regimen changes.

NPH and Lente users. For recreational play, insulin adjustments vary widely depending on the sport. For shorter play, you may need minimal regimen changes. For more prolonged play, you may need to reduce preactivity short-acting insulins by 10 to 50 percent. For power sports in general, you will not need to reduce insulin doses as much as you would need for prolonged endurance sports. In some cases, you will need to increase your insulin dose because of the release of glucose-raising hormones during intense activities. Also, if you take morning doses of NPH or Lente, you may need to reduce them 10 to 30 percent for an afternoon activity. For more prolonged activities, you may need 10 to 30 grams of carbohydrate per hour as well, depending on the reductions in insulin doses. You may need to reduce the insulin dose for meals following the activity by 10 to 20 percent for some sports (for example, a two-hour intense basketball game). For certain sports, you may also reduce bedtime doses of NPH or Lente by 10 to 20 percent following depleting exercise, and you may need an extra bedtime snack.

Insulin pump users. For recreational power sports, insulin adjustments are sport-specific. You may require no insulin or diet changes for easy or brief play. For more prolonged play such as team practices, you may need to reduce preactivity short-acting insulin boluses as well as basal insulin rates during an activity by 10 to 50 percent, depending on intensity and duration of the sport. Insulin reductions,

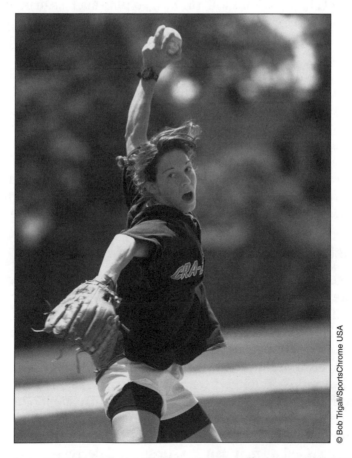

Recreational power sports such as softball may have no effect on your blood sugar or they may actually raise them.

however, are generally smaller than those required for endurance sports due to the intense, brief nature of power activities. In some cases, blood sugar levels may actually increase due to the intensity of the activity, necessitating an increase in insulin rather than a decrease. For more prolonged or intense participation, you may need 10 to 30 grams of carbohydrate per hour, depending on your reductions in insulin basal rates and boluses. You may need to reduce insulin boluses by 10 to 25 percent following certain sports, and you may need an increase in carbohydrate intake or reduce basal insulin rates by 10 to 20 percent after the activity. You may need additional snacks as well.

Ultralente users. For most recreational power sports, insulin adjustments depend on the sport. Short or easy play may require no insulin or diet changes. For more prolonged play such as team practices, you may need to reduce preactivity short-acting insulins by 10 to 50 percent. Insulin reductions, however, are generally smaller than those required for endurance sports due to the intense, brief nature of power activities. In some cases, blood sugar levels may actually increase due to the intensity of the activity, necessitating an increase in insulin rather than a decrease. For more prolonged or intense participation, you may need 10 to 30 grams of carbohydrate per hour, depending on your reductions in insulin and timing with short-acting insulins. For certain sports you may reduce bedtime doses of Ultralente by 10 to 15 percent as well. You may also need a bedtime snack to prevent overnight hypoglycemia following exercise that depletes a substantial amount of muscle glycogen.

Intensity, Duration, and Other Effects

The level of effort, duration, and type of power sport (recreational or more competitive play) have the biggest effects on blood sugar levels. The position you play can also affect the overall effort required. Being more active overall (and thus depleting more muscle glycogen from repeated, powerful movements) can reduce blood sugar levels more dramatically. Recreational play is usually less intense but more prolonged than competitive play. A short, intense competition such as a wrestling match may cause blood sugar levels to rise due to the intensity and brevity of the activity, whereas recreational softball may have no effect on blood sugar levels. Two hours of basketball may cause a substantial decrease in blood sugar levels immediately following the activity and overnight.

BASKETBALL

This court activity involves a lot of stop-and-start movements and quick, powerful moves such as shooting, passing, and dribbling. As a result, it is much more anaerobic in nature than aerobic. However, when you play for an hour or more fairly continuously, substantial muscle glycogen depletion and blood sugar use can occur. Basketball can also have a more aerobic component when athletes run up and down the court at a moderate pace. You may need changes in both insulin and diet to prevent a drop in blood sugar levels during or after a game or practice.

Duration of basketball practice or games and circulating insulin levels during play are what affect blood sugar the most. If you can exercise with minimal levels of insulin (i.e., three to four hours after the last injection of short-acting insulin, early in the morning, or without your insulin pump), you will maintain your blood sugar levels more effectively with a decreased carbohydrate intake. Otherwise, you may need more carbohydrate. If you play for a long time, muscle glycogen repletion following the activity may cause a significant decrease in blood sugar that must be compensated for by increased carbohydrate intake and/or reductions in insulin doses.

Athlete Examples

These real-life examples demonstrate that diet, insulin, or both can be modified to maintain blood sugar control during and following basketball play.

Insulin Changes Alone

An NPH user reduces his morning shot of NPH by 1 unit (from 24 units to 23) and his predinner Humalog by 2 units for one hour of basketball in the evenings. Sometimes his blood sugars still increase while playing basketball and then drop too low following exercise. He decreases his evening Lente by 2 units after prolonged playing.

A pump user disconnects his pump to play basketball. If he plays in the morning, his blood sugars often increase with exercise so he takes a bolus of 1 unit before disconnecting if his starting blood sugar is between 100 and 120 mg/dl.

BASKETBALL

User	Insulin	Diet
NPH/Lente	• Reduce short-acting insulin by 20-50% before playing basketball, depending on expected length of play, starting blood sugar, and desired increase in carbohydrate. • For play in the early morning, short-acting insulin may only need to be reduced by 10-20% due to a higher insulin resistance at that time of day. • Reduce morning doses of NPH or Lente (if taken) by 10-20% for planned afternoon play. • Consider lowering short-acting insulin taken after more strenuous play by 10-20%. • Possibly reduce evening dose of NPH or Lente by 10-25% following extended play.	• Increase carbohydrate intake by 10-25 grams per hour. • Depending on the insulin reductions and starting blood sugar levels, eat up to 15-30 grams of carbohydrate per hour during play. • Early-morning or premeal exercise may need a lesser carbohydrate supplementation. • Consider eating an additional bedtime snack following more strenuous play to reduce the risk for nocturnal hypoglycemia.
Insulin Pump	• Remove your insulin pump or reduce basal rates by 50-75% during the activity. • Reduce preactivity boluses by 25-50% if taken within several hours of playing. • Consider keeping basal rates 10-15% lower for several hours (or even overnight) after strenuous or prolonged play.	• You may need an additional 10-30 grams of carbohydrate per hour, depending on circulating insulin levels and starting blood sugars. • Reduce carbohydrate intake for exercise with lower circulating insulin levels (when the pump is removed, in the early morning, or 3-4 hours after the last bolus of insulin). • Eat a bedtime snack following prolonged activity to reduce the risk of nocturnal hypoglycemia.
Ultralente	• Reduce short-acting insulin doses by 25-50% for play following meals. • For early-morning exercise or when circulating insulin levels are lower (more than 3-4 hours following the last injection of short-acting insulin), any insulin reduction will be less (10-25%). • Consider reducing evening Ultralente doses by 10-15% following extended playing to prevent overnight hypoglycemia.	• Consume an extra 10-30 grams of carbohydrate per hour, depending on circulating insulin levels and starting blood sugars. • Eat an additional snack at bedtime to prevent nocturnal hypoglycemia.

Another pump user disconnects his pump to play for up to two hours. He decreases his usual predinner bolus by 50 percent. Also, the next morning he has to reduce his prebreakfast bolus by 25 percent to avoid hypoglycemia.

Diet Changes Alone

When a bedtime-only NPH user plays basketball for up to 90 minutes in the mornings, he tries to start with a blood sugar around 200 mg/dl by eating extra carbohydrate without taking any additional Humalog. He finds that he is so active while playing that he has to eat a little extra carbohydrate to prevent hypoglycemia even though he plays before lunch, when circulating Humalog is minimal.

Combined Insulin and Diet Changes

For two-hour basketball practices, an NPH user makes changes based on her starting blood sugars. If her blood sugar is high, she takes some Humalog before playing. If low, she eats crackers and juice. Following practice, she may reduce her dinner Humalog by 1 to 2 units if her blood sugars are on the low side. At bedtime, she may reduce her NPH by 1 to 4 units (from 22 units) depending on how active she was.

A pump user checks his blood sugar, eats a snack without bolusing, disconnects his pump, and plays basketball. He will reattach his pump and bolus if his blood sugar rises while playing, but usually his blood sugars stay normal during the 30 minutes or so that he plays.

Intensity, Duration, and Other Effects

Effect of circulating insulin levels. For intense pick-up games of basketball, an NPH user finds that he has trouble playing until most of the Regular insulin from his previous meal is gone from his system.

VOLLEYBALL

This activity involves short, powerful moves (serving or hitting the ball) and is generally anaerobic in nature. Overall energy expenditure can be relatively low, depending on the intensity of play. Volleyball practices may cause greater energy expenditure than volleyball games. Insulin and diet changes will depend on the intensity and duration of play, but you will usually need fewer changes for volleyball compared to more intense and active court sports like basketball.

Intensity of play and circulating insulin levels have the biggest effects on blood sugar levels. Recreational play can involve minimal activity as players are not involved actively in every play, and moving to and hitting the ball require only short bursts of activity. If you can exercise with minimal levels of circulating insulin (three to four hours after the last injection of short-acting insulin, early in the morning, or with a disconnected pump), you will maintain blood sugar levels more effectively with minimal, if any, carbohydrate intake. For more active or prolonged participation, you will need more carbohydrates or insulin changes.

Athlete Examples

The following examples demonstrate that the intensity of play and circulating insulin levels at the time of play can have the greatest effects on the blood sugar response to volleyball participation.

Insulin Changes Alone

For volleyball, an NPH user usually takes only 50 percent of his usual Humalog at the meal preceding the exercise. He drinks juice if needed during the activity. A pump user removes his pump and checks his blood sugar every 30 minutes while playing.

Diet Changes Alone

For one hour of intense volleyball, an NPH user eats 1 to 2 grams extra carbohydrates before playing, depending on her blood glucose levels, and a minimum of 1 gram of carbohydrate afterward regardless of her blood sugar level.

For one hour of moderate-intensity volleyball, a pump user does not adjust his basal rate, but he does consume about 20 grams of extra carbohydrate.

An Ultralente user eats minimal additional carbohydrate as needed for a recreational game of volleyball before dinner. She

VOLLEYBALL

User	Insulin	Diet
NPH/Lente	• Reduce short-acting insulin dose by 10-25% before prolonged or intense play. • For easy recreational activity, make minimal (if any) insulin reductions. • Changes in evening doses of short-acting, NPH, and Lente insulins are usually unnecessary for this activity when done recreationally. • For more intense play, slightly reduce insulin boluses by 10-20% lower afterward.	• Consume an additional 10-20 grams of carbohydrate per hour depending on the insulin reductions and intensity of activity. • Supplement with fewer carbohydrates for early-morning exercise or exercise before meals (when circulating insulin levels are lower).
Insulin Pump	• Consider removing the insulin pump during more active play. • If you keep the insulin pump attached, reduce basal rates by 25-50% during more competitive play. • Reduce preactivity boluses by 10-25% if taken within 2-3 hours of playing. • Resume normal basal insulin rates following recreational play. • For more intense play, slight reductions in insulin boluses (10-20% lower) may be necessary.	• Consume an additional 10-20 grams of carbohydrate per hour, depending on circulating insulin levels and intensity of play. • Exercise when circulating insulin levels are lower (before meals or early in the morning) may require even less carbohydrate intake.
Ultralente	• Decrease short-acting insulins by 10-25% for more strenuous play. • A lesser decrease may be necessary for early-morning exercise or at other times when circulating insulin levels are lower (when no short-acting insulins have been taken for 3-4 hours). • For easy recreational play, make minimal (if any) short-acting insulin reductions.	• Consume an extra 10-20 grams of carbohydrate per hour depending on circulating insulin levels and intensity of activity. • Supplement with less carbohydrate for exercise in the early morning or 3-4 hours following the last injection of short-acting insulin. • Make minimal increases in carbohydrate intake for recreational play.

does not adjust her insulin for games at that time of day. If she plays volleyball after dinner, she eats an extra 10 to 15 grams of carbohydrate with her dinner.

Combined Insulin and Diet Changes

An NPH user decreases her meal Regular dose by 1 to 3 units and then drinks eight to 16 ounces of juice as needed before beginning her exercise. Another NPH user decreases her dose of Regular insulin by 10 percent before playing a game and eats 15 grams of carbohydrate at halftime during the game.

For two-hour practices in the afternoon and tournaments on weekends, another NPH user reduces her morning NPH by up to 50 percent (from 30 units), and she drinks regular soda during the activity as needed.

BASEBALL AND SOFTBALL

These activities usually require only short bursts of movement like sprinting, hitting, and throwing, so they are very anaerobic in nature. As a result, you may not experience much overall energy expenditure. However, these activities do help children participants to improve on their hand-eye coordination and fine motor skills and are very useful for stimulating overall motor development. The total activity experienced during these sports may also depend on the position you play: a catcher or a pitcher may be more active overall than other infielders as either one would be involved with most of the plays. You can make alterations in food or insulin to compensate for the activity, but you may need minimal changes due to the anaerobic nature of these sports.

The level of effort (recreational or competitive), duration, and the position you play will affect blood sugar levels. The catcher and pitcher positions, which require more activity while the defensive team is on the field, require more overall energy expenditure. Continuous activity can decrease blood sugar levels. Recreational play like a softball game can actually be quite sedentary since only one player at a time is up to bat for half the inning, and during the other half, most players are not involved with every play. More competitive play involving conditioning drills during practices will increase the potential glucose-lowering effects of the activity and require greater regimen changes.

Athlete Examples

The following examples show that recreational play may require minimal changes, but more prolonged, intense practices can reduce blood sugars to a greater degree.

BASEBALL AND SOFTBALL*

User	Insulin	Diet
NPH/Lente	• Reduce short-acting insulin by 10-20% prior to more intense or prolonged play such as team practices. • Fewer changes are necessary for exercise when circulating insulin levels are lower (more than 3-4 hours following the last short-acting insulin).	• Increase carbohydrate intake by 5-15 grams depending on the reduction in short-acting insulin for longer play. • Consume 10-30 grams of supplemental carbohydrate for team practices involving interval running and other activities.
Insulin Pump	• Reduce preactivity insulin boluses and basal rates during play by 10-15% for more intense or prolonged play such as team practices. • Basal rate reductions alone may be sufficient to compensate for most activities.	• Increase carbohydrate intake by 5-15 grams for more intense or prolonged play. • Supplement with 10-30 grams of carbohydrate for team practices involving significant running and activity.
Ultralente	• Reduce preactivity short-acting insulin by 10-15% for more intense or prolonged activities such as practices. • When circulating levels of insulin are low (more than 3-4 hours after the last injection of short-acting insulin), reduce preexercise short-acting doses.	• Supplement with 5-15 grams of carbohydrate for intense or prolonged practices. • Supplement with 10-30 grams of carbohydrate for practices involving interval runs or other significant activity.

* For recreational play, most individuals will not need to make any adjustments to diet or insulin.

Diet Changes Alone

An NPH user eats at least 15 extra grams of carbohydrate or more before playing, depending on her blood sugar levels. For a two-hour softball game after dinner, another NPH user usually adds 30 grams of carbohydrate to his dinner and then tests his blood sugar before, during, and after the activity.

Combined Insulin and Diet Changes

For 90 minutes of softball once a week, an NPH user makes no changes in his insulin or food intake. Another NPH user may reduce his Regular insulin up to 1 unit or eat an additional snack of up to 200 calories if needed.

On the afternoons that another NPH user has baseball practice, he does not make any adjustments before his activity, but he decreases his dinner Humalog by 1 unit following practice or games. He keeps juice, regular soda, glucose tablets, and candy available during the activity to treat low blood sugars. At bedtime if his blood sugar is below 90 mg/dl, he eats an additional carbohydrate and protein with his bedtime snack.

A pump user decreases his meal Humalog bolus from 2.0 to 1.7 units if he plans to exercise. He drinks a sport drink 10 to 20 minutes into the activity, and he tries to begin exercise with a blood sugar of 140 mg/dl or above.

Intensity, Duration, and Other Effects

Effect of intensity. A pump user plays softball in the summer and does not adjust her insulin or supplement with food. She finds that sometimes the competitiveness actually causes an increase in her blood sugars.

Effect of position played. For baseball, an insulin pump user may reduce the basal rate on his pump by 30 to 35 percent depending on the length and intensity of the position he plays. When he plays catcher, he decreases the basal rate even more. He drinks sport drinks during the games and occasionally disconnects his pump when his blood sugar is 120 or below.

FIELD HOCKEY

Depending on the position you play, field hockey is a combination of stop-and-start movements and longer sustained runs involving both anaerobic and aerobic components. As such, field hockey participation can result in significant use of both muscle glycogen and blood sugar. It is also most similar to soccer play when compared to endurance sports, and its play can definitely contain an aerobic component. Of course, the position you play will greatly affect the overall level of activity (i.e., goalies will run a lot less than the field players). You may need regimen changes in diet and insulin depending on your position in the game.

Duration, intensity, and levels of circulating insulin affect the blood sugar response to field hockey. Prolonged play will cause greater reductions in muscle glycogen stores and blood sugar levels

FIELD HOCKEY

User	Insulin	Diet
NPH/Lente	• Reduce short-acting insulin doses before breakfast by 20-30% for morning games or practices. • For afternoon practices and games, reduce morning doses of NPH or Lente by 10-25%, or reduce lunchtime short-acting insulin doses by 20-30%. • For practices and games when circulating insulin levels are low (before meals), make fewer regimen changes. • Following prolonged or intense activity, consider reducing doses of short-acting insulin for the next meal by 20-30% and evening doses of NPH or Lente by 10-20%.	• Consume an additional 15-30 grams of carbohydrate per hour depending on insulin reductions and intensity of the activity. • Eat an additional bedtime snack to prevent overnight hypoglycemia.
Insulin Pump	• During any field hockey practice or game, reduce basal rates on the insulin pump by 25-100%, depending on the length and intensity of the activity. • A midfielder running more continuously for an hour-long game may need a larger reduction (50-75%) than a goalie (25%). • Doses of short-acting insulin taken before play can be reduced by 20-40% as well. • Make fewer changes may be necessary when circulating insulin levels are lower (before meals). • Following prolonged or intense play, consider reducing doses of short-acting insulin for the next meal by 20-30% as well as overnight basal insulin rates by 10-15%.	• Depending on the level of activity and insulin reductions, consume 15-30 grams of additional carbohydrate per hour. • Eat an additional bedtime snack to prevent overnight hypoglycemia following prolonged or strenuous play, especially if basal rates are not reduced.
Ultralente	• For field hockey practices and games, decrease doses of short-acting insulin by 20-30%. • Make fewer regimen changes may be necessary when circulating insulin levels are lower (before meals). • Following prolonged or intense games or practices, reduce doses of short-acting insulin for the next meal by 20-30% and/or reduce evening Ultralente doses by 10-15%.	• Depending on the activity and reductions in insulin, consume 15-30 grams of additional carbohydrate per hour. • Consider eating an additional bedtime snack to prevent nocturnal hypoglycemia, especially following prolonged or strenuous play.

and will require a greater carbohydrate intake combined with reductions in insulin both before and after playing. The position largely determines the intensity of play. The position involves either fairly continuous running or just occasional action. A midfielder running more continuously for an hour-long game will need less insulin and more food than a goalie. During practices, activity levels among positions may be more similar if all team members do continuous running or shooting drills. An athlete's level of circulating insulin during field hockey will also determine the need for any extra carbohydrate. If you take short-acting insulins one to two hours before a practice or game, your blood glucose is more likely to decrease than if only basal amounts of insulin are present in the body during practice or a game (i.e., three to four hours after the last injection of short-acting insulin or just before the next meal). During the regular field hockey season, you will need to decrease basal insulin doses (intermediate and long-acting insulins or a pump basal rate) more than during off-season times as well.

Athlete Examples

An insulin pump user plays an hour of field hockey once a week. For this activity, she takes her pump off. When she reconnects it, she gives herself a bolus of 2 units. She does not eat any extra food before playing, but she eats 15 grams of carbohydrate afterward. When playing tournaments, she wears her pump between games.

For practices and games, an Ultralente user may reduce her preworkout Humalog insulin by a couple of units. During the season her Ultralente dose is lower both in the morning and the evening. She eats additional snacks as needed.

LACROSSE

Depending on the position you play, lacrosse is a combination of stop-and-start movements and longer sustained runs (anaerobic and aerobic components). It can result in significant use of both muscle glycogen and blood sugar. Your position will greatly affect the overall level of activity: goaltenders will run a lot less than field players. Field position will determine regimen changes in diet and insulin. For general and specific recommendations for a comparable sport, refer to the "Field Hockey" section in this chapter.

AMERICAN FOOTBALL AND RUGBY

These sports are very anaerobic in nature. Most football plays last only 10 to 20 seconds, and power moves occur during plays: pushing on the offensive or defensive line, throwing the ball, sprinting into position, running powerfully with the ball, or blocking. Practices may vary in the types of activities and are more prolonged overall, causing potentially greater reductions in blood sugar than games, especially if the usual position you play during games is that of benchwarmer. The position you play and whether the activity is a practice or a game will determine changes in insulin or food intake. With more recreational play in these sports, running tends to be more emphasized but play is less intense and shorter, necessitating fewer regimen changes.

Different factors will affect the blood sugar response to these sports. The position you play can greatly affect the type of activity you do. Players in positions that require more running (wide receiver, running back, defensive back) may use muscle glycogen differently than players in "brute force" positions (offensive and defensive linemen) who just block and do truly anaerobic work during plays. More running may reduce blood sugars during the activity, but muscle glycogen repletion following the activity may require a greater carbohydrate intake or reduction in insulin for all players following the activity. Practices and games differ in energy expenditure and blood glucose levels. Practices tend to involve more prolonged play and may cause a greater fall in blood sugars than game situations. Preseason practices, especially twice daily, will also cause greater regimen changes than shorter, easier practices during the regular season, especially before an upcoming game. For more recreational play in these sports, running tends to be more emphasized, but play is usually less intense and shorter, necessitating smaller regimen changes.

Athlete Examples

These examples show that recreational play requires quite different regimen changes than collegiate or more competitive play.

Diet Changes Alone

For English rugby practices and games, an NPH user increases his carbohydrate intake after practice or games. Before practice,

AMERICAN FOOTBALL AND RUGBY

User	Insulin	Diet
NPH/Lente	• For afternoon practices, reduce morning NPH or Lente doses by 25-50% for 2- to 3-hour practice sessions, or reduce short-acting lunch doses by 25-50%. • Reduce insulin doses by 10-30% for shorter or less intense practices. • For practicing when circulating insulin levels are lower (before dinner when no morning NPH is taken), make minimal reductions in insulin doses for the prior meal. • Reduce predinner (short-acting) and evening or bedtime insulin (NPH or Lente) by 10-30% following prolonged or intense practice sessions or games.	• Consume 15-45 grams of carbohydrate per hour depending on insulin reductions and practice intensity. • Consume additional carbohydrate to prevent later-onset hypoglycemia.
Insulin Pump	• For afternoon practice sessions of 2-3 hours, reduce basal insulin rates by 25-50%. • If you remove the pump completely for that length of time, check blood sugars at least hourly and reconnect the pump and bolus as needed to correct for any significant rise in blood sugars. • Reduce the premeal insulin bolus by 25-50% for practices or games within 2-3 hours following that meal. • For shorter or less intense practices or when 3-4 hours after the last insulin bolus, make more minimal reductions in insulin boluses at preceding meals. • Make minimal changes in insulin doses for practicing (3-4 hours after the last bolus), when circulating insulin levels are lower. • Basal rates should remain 10-20% lower (and possibly overnight) for several hours following intense or prolonged practices or games. • Reduce predinner insulin boluses by 10-30% after strenuous play to prevent later-onset hypoglycemia.	• Consume 15-45 grams of carbohydrate per hour depending on insulin reductions and practice intensity. • Consume additional carbohydrate after play and possibly at bedtime to prevent later-onset hypoglycemia, depending on insulin reductions.

User	Insulin	Diet
Ultralente	• For afternoon practices of 2-3 hours, reduce morning Ultralente doses by 0-25%. • Reduce prelunch short-acting insulin dose by 25-50% depending on changes in carbohydrate intake. • For practices when circulating insulin levels are lower (3-4 hours after the last injection of short-acting insulin), make minimal reductions in insulin at the preceding meal. • Reduce predinner insulin by 10-30% following prolonged or intense practice sessions or games to prevent later-onset hypoglycemia.	• Supplement with 15-45 grams of carbohydrate per hour depending on insulin reductions and practice intensity. • For shorter or less intense practices, make minimal reductions in insulin or minimal increases in carbohydrate intake. • Eat additional carbohydrate as necessary during and after the activity (and possibly at bedtime) to prevent hypoglycemia.

his circulating insulin levels from his morning NPH and Regular are minimal because his practices are from 6:30 to 8:00 P.M. He takes his evening insulin and eats dinner after practice. He needs to eat more after practices than after games as they are more prolonged and intense.

Combined Insulin and Diet Changes

An NPH user participated in collegiate football. For summer preseason practice (twice daily for three hours at a time), he cut his NPH by 5 units (from 8 to 3) in the morning and took no Regular insulin (he usually took 2 units). He drank a sport drink during practice and ate candy as needed. He used to test his blood sugar 20 to 30 times a day. In doing that, he found that a blood sugar of 180 mg/dl and rising allowed him to practice without becoming hypoglycemic. He also cut his bedtime NPH by 1 unit (from 8 to 7 units). For practice during the season (five days a week for three hours) and one game on the weekend, he still cut back on his morning NPH by 3 units but took 1 unit of Regular. He tested his blood sugar before practice and ate 15 to 30 grams of carbohydrate as necessary. His dinner and bedtime doses returned to normal, as the practices were less intense than during preseason.

For rugby practices and games, another NPH user reduces his short-acting insulin by 1 to 2 units before playing and eats more carbohydrates as needed. He keeps juice and chocolate bars available during this activity. For recreational flag football, a pump user suspends his pump while playing and drinks a sport drink as needed to maintain his blood sugar levels.

GYMNASTICS

Gymnastics requires mainly short, powerful movements both during practice and competition. Few aspects of this sport are aerobic or prolonged. Most energy is supplied through immediate sources (ATP and CP) and other anaerobic sources (muscle glycogen and the lactic acid system). Prolonged practices can result in reduced blood glucose levels, but most gymnastics activities may require minimal changes in diet and insulin due to the short, intense nature of most gymnastics routines.

The duration of gymnastics participation has the greatest effect on blood sugar levels. Doing several short routines during a gymnastics meet may have minimal effects. Two to three hours of practice will have more of a glucose-lowering effect due to the greater total activity and use of muscle glycogen.

Athlete Examples

An NPH user participates in gymnastics eight to 14 hours per week. She increases her carbohydrate intake before and after practice but does not modify her insulin; she only takes insulin before breakfast and dinner (NPH and Regular).

GYMNASTICS

User	Insulin	Diet
NPH/Lente	• For afternoon practices, reduce morning NPH or Lente (if taken) by 10-20%. • Decrease short-acting insulin doses by 10-20% if the activity follows a meal. • Keep evening doses of NPH or Lente the same. For exceptionally strenuous practices, consider reducing evening doses by 10-20%.	• Increase carbohydrate intake by 10-25 grams per hour for extended gymnastics practices depending on circulating insulin levels. • Make minimal carbohydrate increases for exercise more than 3-4 hours after the last meal. • Eat an additional bedtime snack following strenuous practices.
Insulin Pump	• Decrease basal insulin rates by 10-50% during gymnastics practice depending on the intensity and duration of the activity. • Remove the pump completely during short routines. • If the pump is removed for longer periods, monitor blood sugars closely and reattach the pump to administer boluses if blood sugars begin to rise significantly. • Consider reducing insulin boluses by 10-20% for gymnastics activity following a meal as well. • Reduce overnight basal insulin rates by 10-15% following especially prolonged or strenuous practices.	• Increase carbohydrate intake by 5-15 grams per hour for extended gymnastics activity depending on insulin changes. • Make minimal carbohydrate increases when insulin levels are reduced, such as 3-4 hours following the last insulin bolus. • Eat an extra bedtime snack (if basal insulin is not reduced) following exceptionally strenuous or prolonged practices.
Ultralente	• If the activity follows a meal, reduce short-acting insulin doses by 10-15%. • Keep Ultralente doses the same unless practices are unusually long and strenuous. In those cases, consider reducing evening doses by 10-20% to prevent noctural hypoglycemia.	• Increase carbohydrate intake by 5-15 grams per hour for extended gymnastics activity. • Make minimal increases in carbohydrate intake for reduced insulin levels or if gymnastics practice occurs when circulating levels of insulin are low (3-4 hours after the last injection of short-acting insulin). • Eat an extra bedtime snack following exceptionally strenuous or prolonged practices.

TRACK AND FIELD

Most track and field events are short, requiring either a near-maximal muscular contraction (like throwing a shot put) or near-maximal full body effort (like long-jumping or sprinting). These types of events use only anaerobic energy sources. Longer track events such as 800-meter runs require more energy production from the lactic acid system and are still primarily anaerobic events. Runs lasting longer than two minutes will begin to utilize a greater proportion of aerobic sources of energy. Track practices may involve running longer distances or repeated intervals and may be more aerobic in nature than track meets where athletes run shorter distances. Changes in insulin or diet are determined more by the duration of aerobic activities and are less affected by anaerobic events.

Blood sugars may tend to decrease more following track practices or meets when muscle glycogen is restored than during practices or meets. The intensity and brevity of events during competitions should allow for fairly easy maintenance of blood sugar levels. You may need more regimen changes to maintain blood sugar levels both during and after practice because of the prolonged activity (compared with meets).

Athlete Examples

These examples demonstrate the usual types of regimen changes required for track and field practices and meets.

Insulin Changes Alone

An Ultralente user usually makes no adjustments to her insulin for track and field workouts and meets. During the season she reduces her Ultralente dose both in the morning and the evening, however. She eats additional snacks as needed.

Diet Changes Alone

An Ultralente user feels her best when she begins track practice at a blood sugar of 120 mg/dl. If her blood sugar is lower, she has a granola bar, sport drink, or juice. She does not adjust her insulin before practice as it is in the late afternoon when circulating insulin levels are lower.

TRACK AND FIELD

User	Insulin	Diet
NPH/Lente	• For afternoon practices, reduce morning NPH or Lente (if taken) by 10-20%. • Reduce short-acting insulin doses by 10-20% as well if the activity follows a meal. • Blood sugars will stay more stable when the activity occurs more than 3-4 hours after the last injection of short-acting insulin. • Make minimal regimen changes for competitive meets due to the brief, intense nature of most events.	• Make minimal increases in carbohydrate intake for short, intense activities. • Increase carbohydrate intake by 10-15 grams per hour for extended practices.
Insulin Pump	• Decrease basal insulin rates by 10-50% during practices, depending on the intensity and duration of the activity. • During short events, remove the pump completely. • Reattach the pump to administer boluses if blood sugars begin to rise significantly after it has been off for more than an hour. • Reduce short-acting insulin doses by 10-20% for track and field activity following a meal as well. • Make minimal regimen changes for competitive meets, as the activity is short and intense in nature.	• Make minimal carbohydrate increases for short, intense activities. • Increase carbohydrate intake by 10-15 grams per hour for extended practices, depending on insulin reductions.
Ultralente	• If the activity follows a meal, reduce short-acting insulin doses by 10-20%. • Make minimal regimen changes for competitive meets, as the events are short and intense in nature.	• Make minimal carbohydrate increases if insulin levels are reduced or practices occur when circulating levels of insulin are low. • Increase carbohydrate intake by 10-15 grams per hour for extended practices, if needed.

Combined Insulin and Diet Changes

For two-hour practices in the afternoon and meets, an NPH user reduces her morning NPH by up to 50 percent (from 30 units). She drinks regular soda during practices as needed. She may also reduce her Regular insulin by 1 unit.

ICE HOCKEY

Ice hockey involves a lot of short power moves such as shooting the puck and skating quickly to another position. The activity can be intense, however, resulting in the use of a significant amount of muscle glycogen as well as blood sugar when you play for an extended period of time. Changes in insulin and diet will be necessary depending on the intensity and duration of play. Practices may require more changes due to their prolonged, less intense nature compared with hockey games. A confounding variable is that ice hockey competitions and practices often occur at unusual times (early-morning practices, late-evening games).

Circulating insulin levels during games or practice affect blood sugar levels. If you can exercise with minimal circulating insulin levels (three to four hours after the last injection of short-acting insulin, early in the morning, or with a disconnected insulin pump), you will more effectively maintain blood sugar levels with a reduced carbohydrate intake. Otherwise, you will need a greater carbohydrate intake. If you play for a long time, the ensuing muscle glycogen repletion may also cause a drop in blood sugar that must be replenished by increased carbohydrate intake and/or reductions in insulin doses.

Athlete Examples

These real-life scenarios show that the varied times of day for ice hockey participation can affect necessary regimen changes.

Insulin Changes Alone

For 60 to 90 minutes of hockey, an NPH user decreases his Humalog insulin by 40 percent before the exercise. He may also limit the amount of NPH he takes before the exercise and add another shot with NPH after the exercise.

Combined Insulin and Diet Changes

An NPH user participates in both practices and hockey games. He usually decreases his insulin dose and drinks a sport drink during the games, then drinks one to two cans of Sport Boost after exercise.

ICE HOCKEY

User	Insulin	Diet
NPH/Lente	• Reduce either morning NPH or Lente or lunchtime short-acting insulin by 25-50% for activity in the afternoon. • Reduce predinner insulin by a similar amount for evening play. • Reduce preexercise insulin by 10-25% for hockey in the early morning. • Following extended play later in the day, reduce evening dose of NPH or Lente by 10-25% as well.	• Consume an additional 15-30 grams of carbohydrate per hour depending on insulin reductions. • Eat a lesser amount of carbohydrates for exercise early in the morning or before meals. • Eat an additional bedtime snack to reduce the risk of nocturnal hypoglycemia, especially after prolonged play later in the day.
Insulin Pump	• Remove the insulin pump or reduce basal rates by 50-75% during the activity. • Reduce preactivity boluses by 25-50% if taken within 2-3 hours of playing. • Reduce basal rates by 10-20% overnight following extended play later in the day.	• Consume an additional 15-30 grams of carbohydrate per hour depending on circulating insulin levels and exercise intensity. • Reduce carbohydrate intake for exercise done when circulating insulin levels are lower (before meals or early in the morning). • A bedtime snack following prolonged activity reduces the risk of nocturnal hypoglycemia.
Ultralente	• Decrease short-acting insulins by 25-50% for activity after meals. • Make lesser reductions in insulin doses for early-morning exercise. • Following extended playing, consider reducing the evening dose of Ultralente by 10-15%.	• Consume an extra 15-30 grams of carbohydrate per hour depending on circulating insulin levels and exercise intensity. • Lower carbohydrate intake for activity in the early morning or several hours following the last injection of short-acting insulin. • Consider eating an additional snack at bedtime to help prevent nighttime hypoglycemia.

Intensity, Duration, and Other Effects

An NPH user varies his management depending on the time of day he exercises and whether it is a game or a practice; he finds that playing hockey intensely at certain times causes his blood sugar levels to increase. If either type of activity shortly follows a meal (within two hours), he decreases his premeal short-acting insulin by a couple of units. If he plays a late game (9:00 P.M.), he keeps his predinner insulin the same but reduces his bedtime NPH by as much as 7 units. For an early and a late game (5:00 P.M. and 9:00 P.M.), he reduces both his premeal short-acting insulin and his bedtime NPH by 5 units. For an evening practice, he only reduces his bedtime NPH by 2 to 3 units.

Effect of time of day. Another NPH user makes adjustments to his insulin intake for hockey according to his blood sugars and the time he plays. For early-morning hockey practices lasting 75 minutes, he decreases his bedtime NPH by 3 units (from 16 to 13 units). He tests his blood sugar before practice and may take 1 to 5 units of Humalog if his blood sugar is high. If his blood sugar is less than 160 mg/dl, he eats a small breakfast before practice, then eats his usual breakfast following practice, making adjustments with Humalog if necessary. If he plays during midmorning or midafternoon, he follows his usual regimen without changing insulin doses. If he plays hockey at dinnertime, he has a light snack before and eats dinner afterward, making adjustments with Humalog at mealtime. For hockey late in the evening, he may reduce his predinner Humalog dose, eat his usual bedtime snack, and reduce his bedtime NPH by 3 units. For a hockey tournament with an erratic schedule, he decreases both his NPH and Humalog doses to accommodate games, tests his blood sugar more frequently, and eats more carbohydrate.

WATER POLO

Water polo usually involves a combination of aerobic activity and anaerobic sprints, especially during competitions. Overall, this sport is more aerobically demanding as it requires constant motion in the water to stay afloat. You will encounter the anaerobic component when play shifts from one end of the pool to the other, requiring a higher-intensity sprint, or when you throw the ball. Training for water polo often focuses on distance swimming as well as shorter sprints. For recommended insulin and diet changes, refer to the section on swimming in chapter 7 and focus on the more intensive swimming recommendations and athlete examples.

POWERLIFTING

This activity depends on short-term energy sources such as phosphates for maximal moves lasting no more than 10 seconds. Powerlifting competitions themselves generally have a minimal impact on blood sugar regulation. The more prolonged training for these events is similar to high-resistance weight training. Increases in muscle mass resulting from this training, though, can greatly increase overall insulin sensitivity and require that insulin doses be lowered. For regimen changes, especially those for higher-intensity workouts, refer to the section on weight training in chapter 9.

WRESTLING

This activity requires short, powerful muscle contractions and is almost purely anaerobic in nature. Wrestling practices may affect blood sugar levels more than competitive meets due to the brevity of competitions. Wrestling bouts are short but they are very intense. A wrestling competition may require few regimen changes to maintain blood sugars. A longer training session may require greater changes, even though most training is intense due to the cumulative effects of repeated bouts of short-intensity activity.

Athlete Examples

An NPH user participates in NCAA Division I college wrestling. During the season, he practices six days a week for two to three hours a day. He finds that he must reduce his preactivity combined Humalog and Regular insulin dose by 2 to 3 units and eat more carbohydrate as determined by his starting blood sugar levels.

For wrestling, a pump user disconnects his pump. He decreases his preexercise meal Humalog bolus from 2 to 1.7 units and has a sport drink 10 to 20 minutes into the activity. He tries to begin exercise with a blood sugar of 140 mg/dl or above.

Many individuals with diabetes participate in power sports, from the recreational softball player to the competitive college basketball player to the professional football athlete. With some consideration about the intensity and duration of your participation, you too can learn to effectively manage your blood sugar levels while enjoying power sports.

WRESTLING

User	Insulin	Diet
NPH/Lente	• Make minimal changes in insulin for participation in wrestling matches (short, intense activity). • Reduce short-acting insulin by 10-20% prior to longer practices. • Reduce morning doses of NPH or Lente by a similar amount for an afternoon practice session. • Consider making a reduction of 10-20% in bedtime NPH doses following long or strenuous practices.	• Increase carbohydrate intake by 15 grams per hour for longer practices. • Consider eating a snack (with 10-15 grams of carbohydrate) before an afternoon practice as well as extra carbohydrate afterward. • Eat a bedtime snack to prevent overnight hypoglycemia following more extended workouts.
Insulin Pump	• Blood sugars during wrestling competitions may be effectively maintained simply by removing the insulin pump during the match. • Longer practices may require a 10-20% reduction in insulin boluses. • Remove insulin pump for long practices, or reduce basal rates by 25-50% during and for up to 1-2 hours following the practice. • If the pump is removed and blood sugars increase, reconnect and bolus with a small amount of insulin periodically. • Give less insulin for food eaten following a strenuous exercise (10-20% less). • Following especially glycogen-depleting workouts, consider lowering overnight basal rates by a small amount (10-15%).	• Increase carbohydrate intake by up to 15 grams per hour for this activity. • Eat additional carbohydrate for the following meal to prevent later-onset hypoglycemia. • Consider eating an extra bedtime snack following more extended workouts.
Ultralente	• Make minimal changes in insulin for participation in wrestling matches as blood sugars are better maintained during short, intense activity. • Reduce short-acting insulin doses by 10-20% for longer practices. • If practices are prolonged, make an additional reduction of 10-20% in short-acting insulin for the following meal. • No Ultralente changes are usually necessary for usual exercise. Following especially strenuous or prolonged workouts, consider reducing evening doses by 10-15%.	• Increase carbohydrate intake by up to 15 grams per hour for this activity, depending on circulating insulin levels. • Additional carbohydrate intake for the following meal and at bedtime may also help prevent nocturnal hypogly-cemia.

Chapter 9

Fitness Activities

If you are reading this chapter, then you must be part of the fitness craze! Whether you participate in aerobic dance classes, learn martial arts, pump up with weights, or push your limits on the StairMaster, you are not alone. We all want an athletic, toned, fit look, and most of us know we have to sweat some to get it. Being physically fit has many health benefits to all people and additional benefits to people with diabetes; these benefits are described in chapter 1. Having diabetes should be your excuse to exercise regularly, not your excuse to be a couch potato! So get out there and get fit! You can participate in most of the activities listed in this chapter in a health club or fitness gym. These activities include aerobic dance and step aerobics, water aerobics, various aerobic conditioning machines (treadmill, StairMaster, elliptical strider, stationary cycle, NordicTrack, and rowing machine), walking and racewalking, weight and resistance circuit training, martial arts (karate, judo, taekwondo, and t'ai chi), boxing, kickboxing, and yoga and stretching.

Fitness activities vary widely with regard to the energy systems recruited and fuels used. Aerobic dance is mainly an aerobic activity, but it may also contain elements of muscular toning and strengthening as well as stretching. Some martial arts may involve only short, intense movements. Aerobic conditioning machines such as stationary cycles or rowing machines provide aerobic and anaerobic conditioning, depending on the intensity and duration of the activity. For a fuller explanation of the various energy systems and energy sources used for different types of exercise, refer to chapter 2.

GENERAL RECOMMENDATIONS

This chapter gives general recommendations for fitness activities. For each specific activity, general recommendations for that type of exercise as well as real-life examples of some people's specific changes in insulin and diet are listed according to their insulin regimen (NPH and Lente, insulin pump, and Ultralente users). *Users of oral hypoglycemic agents are not listed separately, but you can use the general recommendations for diet changes alone (or those specifically for NPH and Lente users) as an approximate guide when blood sugars are in a normal range.* When blood sugars are elevated, you will need to reduce your dietary intake. Regular participation in fitness activities can cause you to lose fat weight, gain muscle mass, and improve your blood sugar control. You may find that these changes in your body will improve your insulin sensitivity and necessitate lower doses of insulin or oral medications. While insulin can be reduced according to some of these guidelines fairly easily, you should make adjustments in oral doses of medication under the advice of a physician only. For more information about the actions of various types of insulins and oral hypoglycemic agents, refer to chapter 3.

The activities included in this section run the gamut from low-intensity activities such as yoga to intense, brief activities such as heavy weight training or kickboxing to endurance activities such as racewalking or stationary cycling. The majority of these, however, are endurance activities utilizing the aerobic oxygen system.

General Insulin and Diet Changes

NPH and Lente users. You will need to reduce your short-acting insulin dose by 10 to 50 percent for most endurance-related fitness activities closely following a meal, depending on the intensity and duration of the activity. You will also need to increase your carbohydrate intake by 10 to 30 grams per hour, depending on the insulin reductions. If you take NPH in the morning, you may reduce that dose of NPH by 10 to 30 percent for exercise in the afternoon and/or eat a carbohydrate snack of 10 to 15 grams. If you exercise when circulating insulin levels are low (three to four hours following the last injection of short-acting insulin, especially when you take NPH or Lente at bedtime only), small increases in carbohydrate intake alone may suffice without insulin reductions. Changes in bedtime doses of NPH are usually not necessary for most of these activities. Minimal changes are necessary for weight training or stretching.

Insulin pump users. Reductions in basal insulin rates of 25 to 100 percent during many of these activities will prevent low blood sugars and possibly the need for an additional carbohydrate intake. For exercise following a meal, you may reduce your meal bolus by 10 to 50 percent and reduce the basal rate during the activity, depending on the intensity and duration of the activity and the desired carbohydrate increase. You may also need to increase your carbohydrate consumption by 10 to 30 grams per hour or more if you do not make appropriate insulin reductions. You may not need changes in basal rates overnight following fitness activities. These recommendations would not apply to most weight training or stretching activities because they require minimal regimen changes.

Ultralente users. You can generally reduce short-acting insulin doses by 10 to 50 percent preceding these activities when they closely follow a meal as well as increase your carbohydrate intake by 10 to 30 grams per hour, depending on the insulin reductions. For later exercise (more than three to four hours after the last short-acting insulin injection), you may need no changes in insulin and only small increases in carbohydrate intake (up to 15 additional grams) due to lower circulating insulin levels. You usually do not need changes in Ultralente doses following these activities. You may need no adjustments for weight training or stretching.

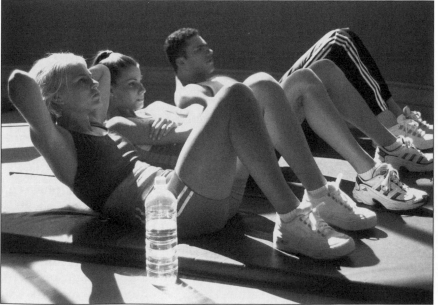

© Nova Stock/International Stock

Aerobic classes are a great way to gain cardiovascular fitness and muscle endurance.

Intensity, Duration, and Other Effects

Exercise intensity and duration, the time of day you exercise, and your starting blood sugar levels have the biggest effects on blood sugar response to fitness activities. Longer workouts will generally have more of a glucose-reducing effect than shorter workouts and may require greater regimen changes to prevent hypoglycemia during and following the activity. High-intensity activities may initially maintain blood sugar levels more effectively, but delayed-onset hypoglycemia is a greater risk due to the muscle glycogen repletion following the activity. Any activity you do early in the morning when insulin resistance is higher will be less likely to reduce blood sugars than exercise after a meal with a short-acting insulin injection or during an insulin peak (such as exercise in the afternoon if you take morning NPH doses). Any activity you do more than three to four hours following the last injection of short-acting insulin (only two to three hours for Humalog insulin) may require minimal changes in insulin or food intake to compensate if no insulins are peaking then. Pump users can most easily achieve lower circulating levels of insulin during the activity by reducing their basal rate of insulin. Starting blood sugar levels will also affect changes in insulin or food intakes. Higher starting levels may actually necessitate an additional injection of short-acting insulin to reduce your blood sugar levels, whereas lower starting levels may increase your need for carbohydrate supplementation.

AEROBIC DANCE AND STEP AEROBICS

These activities are mainly aerobic in nature, with periods of greater intensity (aerobic portion) and lesser intensity (stretching and toning portions). Using small weights and repetitions (such as abdominal work) during the activity still results in mainly aerobic workouts due to the prolonged nature of the exercise and the emphasis on muscular endurance over strength. Classes will also vary in intensity based on individual effort and participation as well as the nature of the class (high-impact, low-impact, step, hip-hop, and others).

Exercise intensity, the time of day you exercise, and starting blood sugar levels have the biggest effects on your blood sugar response to aerobic dance and step aerobics. Higher-intensity workouts will generally reduce blood sugar more than lower-intensity aerobics and require greater regimen changes to prevent hypoglycemia.

AEROBIC DANCE AND STEP AEROBICS

User	Insulin	Diet
NPH/Lente	• Reduce short-acting insulin doses by 25-50% for exercise following within several hours of a meal. • Reduce morning NPH doses by 20-30% for exercise in the afternoon (if taken), or reduce the short-acting insulin taken for lunch by a similar or greater amount. • For exercise when circulating insulin levels are lower (before meals or early in the morning), make lesser reductions (if any) in insulin. • You will usually not need to make reductions in bedtime doses of NPH.	• Increase carbohydrate intake by 10-25 grams per hour, depending on insulin reductions. • For exercise when circulating insulin levels are lower (before meals or early in the morning), increase carbohydrate intake minimally.
Insulin Pump	• Reduce basal insulin rates by 50-100% during aerobics; doing so may eliminate the need for any additional carbohydrates. • Consider making basal rate reductions 30-60 minutes before the exercise and maintain at a lower level for 1-2 hours following exercise to further reduce the need for any supplemental carbohydrates. • For exercise more closely following a meal, reduce the insulin bolus by 25-50% as well depending on the intensity of the activity. • Changes in overnight basal rates are usually not necessary following this activity.	• Increase carbohydrate consumption by up to 10-20 grams per hour, depending on insulin reductions. • If insulin levels are lowered sufficiently to reduce circulating insulin levels during the activity, then increase carbohydrate intake minimally.
Ultralente	• Reduce short-acting insulins by 25-50% for exercise following a meal. • For exercise when circulating insulin levels are lower (before meals or early in the morning), make lesser reductions (if any) in short-acting insulin. • You should not need to reduce Ultralente doses to prevent overnight hypoglycemia.	• Increase carbohydrate consumption by 10-20 grams per hour depending on the actual reductions in insulin. • For exercise more than 3-4 hours after the last short-acting insulin injection, increase carbohydrate intake immediately before aerobics (if needed) instead of reducing insulin at the previous meal to prevent preexercise hyperglycemia. • With lower circulating insulin levels during the activity, increase carbohydrate intake minimally.

Early-morning aerobics (before breakfast, when insulin resistance is higher) will be less likely to reduce blood sugars than exercise following a short-acting insulin injection or during an NPH insulin peak. You will need minimal changes in insulin or food intake if you do aerobics more than three to four hours following the last injection of short-acting insulin, especially if you take NPH at bedtime only or if you take Ultralente. If you are a pump user, you can most easily achieve minimal circulating levels of insulin during the activity by reducing the basal rate of insulin. Starting blood sugar levels will also affect changes in insulin or food intakes. Higher starting levels may actually necessitate an additional injection of short-acting insulin to decrease blood sugar levels, whereas lower starting levels may increase the need for carbohydrate supplementation, especially closely following a meal.

Athlete Examples

These real-life examples show the variety of regimen changes that you can use if you participate in aerobics classes. The type of class you take largely affects the adjustments you need, exercise timing, and starting blood sugars.

Insulin Changes Alone

For 60 minutes of aerobics, flexibility, and strength training, a pump user decreases the basal rate on her pump by 50 percent for one hour before the activity until one hour after. She only eats an extra snack if she has low blood sugar. For 60 minutes of aerobics, another pump user decreases her preexercise meal bolus by 25 to 50 percent and decreases her basal rate by 50 to 75 percent while exercising, depending on the intensity of the class.

Another pump user decreases her basal rate one hour before doing step aerobics and keeps it reduced (down to 0.2 units per hour, a 50 percent decrease from her usual) until two hours after she finishes exercising. She also keeps orange juice and glucose tablets nearby during the activity in case of hypoglycemia.

Diet Changes Alone

An NPH user eats extra carbohydrate before 60 minutes of aerobics or step aerobics. She finds that her blood sugar needs to be

200 mg/dl before the class to avoid hypoglycemia during the activity since she does not adjust her insulin.

A pump user usually eats extra carbohydrate before and after 60 to 90 minutes of low-impact or step aerobics. Her aerobics classes are not around meal times, so she does not adjust her premeal Humalog bolus.

Combined Insulin and Diet Changes

For 50 minutes of intense aerobic dance, an NPH user (morning and bedtime) decreases either her Humalog or NPH by 20 to 30 percent, depending on which insulin is active close to the time she does this activity. She also consumes an extra 15 grams of carbohydrate before exercising if her blood sugar is less than 120 mg/dl, unless the exercise is right after a meal.

A pump user decreases her meal bolus of Humalog by 50 percent if she does Jazzercise after a meal and suspends her pump for 30 to 40 minutes during the exercise. If she does not do her activity after a meal, she decreases the basal rate on her pump by 50 percent, eats a snack if her starting blood sugar is 120 mg/dl or less, and supplements with 10 to 15 grams (more if needed) of carbohydrate for each hour of exercise.

Another pump user disconnects her pump during step aerobics. If her blood sugar is high at the start, she may take a bolus of 1 unit for every 100 mg/dl over normal before disconnecting. Her carbohydrate to insulin intake before exercising is 50 grams for a 1-unit bolus of Humalog and 20 grams for 1 unit for six hours after exercise.

An Ultralente user teaches aerobics and step aerobics. For these intense 60-minute classes, she reduces her Humalog by 50 percent at the meal before the exercise and drinks carbohydrate fluids during the classes.

Intensity, Duration, and Other Effects

Effect of time of day. An NPH user does aerobics early in the morning before her breakfast and morning dose of NPH and Humalog. She finds that she does not need to ingest any extra food due to the time of day and lack of insulin. If she exercises later in the day, she drinks some juice or eats a snack before exercising.

Effect of initial blood sugars. An NPH user leads 60-minute high-intensity step interval classes with weights. Before class she will sometimes take an additional 1 to 2 units of Humalog as her blood sugars tend to run higher in the late afternoon. If her blood sugar is less than 200 mg/dl, she will not usually take any insulin. If it is more than 200, she takes the Humalog before starting so that her blood sugar is in a normal range at the end of class.

WATER AEROBICS

This activity is similar to aerobic dance except for its intensity. Workouts in the pool are not weight-bearing like regular aerobics; usually they are less intense. You also place less stress on the lower limb joints. It is still aerobic in nature, utilizing fats and carbohydrates, with periods of greater and lesser intensity. A workout will also vary in intensity based on individual effort and participation.

The time of day you exercise and the circulating insulin levels during the activity have the biggest effects on your blood sugar response to water aerobics. If you do water aerobics early in the morning when insulin resistance is higher, you will be less likely to reduce blood sugars than if you exercise after an insulin injection or during an insulin peak. If you do water aerobics more than three to four hours following the last injection of short-acting insulin, you may require minimal changes in insulin or food intake, especially if you take NPH at bedtime only and if you use Ultralente. If you use an insulin pump, you can most easily achieve circulating levels of insulin during the activity by reducing the basal rate of insulin or disconnecting the pump during the activity.

Athlete Examples

A pump user disconnects her pump during 60 minutes of water aerobics and activities that she does before lunch. She effectively maintains her blood sugar during the activity without any supplemental carbohydrate.

AEROBIC CONDITIONING MACHINES

Exercises on the treadmill, StairMaster, elliptical strider, stationary cycle, NordicTrack, and rowing machine are all aerobic in nature because they are sustained for more than two minutes. These activi-

WATER AEROBICS

User	Insulin	Diet
NPH/Lente	• Reduce short-acting insulin doses by 15-40% for exercise within several hours after a meal. • Reduce morning NPH doses by 10-30% for afternoon exercise if no short-acting insulin is taken for lunch. • You should not need to reduce in bedtime doses of NPH.	• Increase carbohydrate intake by 10-15 grams per hour, depending on insulin reductions. • For exercise when circulating insulin levels are lower, consume carbohydrates at 0-10 grams per hour.
Insulin Pump	• Remove the insulin pump altogether, or reduce the basal rate by 25-50% during water aerobics (as long as the pump is waterproof). • For exercise following a meal, reduce both the insulin bolus and basal rate during the activity by 15-40%. • Keep overnight basal rates the same following this activity.	• Increase carbohydrate consumption by 10-15 grams per hour, depending on insulin bolus and basal rate reductions. • Consume less carbohydrate intake may be needed when this activity is done when circulating insulin levels are lower (like before meals).
Ultralente	• Decrease short-acting insulin preceding this activity by 15-40% when water aerobics follow a meal. • You should not need to make changes in Ultralente doses.	• Increase carbohydrate consumption by 10-15 grams per hour when insulin is not reduced much. • For exercise more than 3-4 hours after the last short-acting insulin, increase carbohydrate intake by less (0-10 grams) for water aerobics.

ties can be quite intense as they generally involve either large muscle groups in the legs or full-body musculature. Some also provide a significant proportion of upper-body work (e.g., NordicTrack and rowing machine). Insulin and diet changes depend primarily on the intensity and duration of the conditioning activity as well as the timing of the exercise.

Treadmill walking or running is similar to walking, racewalking, or running outdoors in terms of the blood sugar response. The only differences arise from environmental conditions that may increase the energy cost of the activity when done outdoors in excessively hot, cold, or windy conditions (refer to walking in this chapter, running in chapter 7, and exercise under environmental extremes in chapter 10).

Sprinting up stadium steps is more anaerobic than using a StairMaster or stair climber, an activity that is essentially a continuous aerobic activity. While the intensity of stair climbing varies with the program you choose (hills, manual, random, and so on), blood sugars will respond mainly to the duration of the activity because stair climbing generally provides higher-level aerobic workouts. Short-duration stair climbing will require minimal changes in insulin and food intake to maintain blood sugars. A longer-duration activity will use more muscle glycogen and other fuels and require greater regimen changes.

Elliptical striders give a workout that is a cross between treadmill and stair climbing exercise. While usually more intense than treadmill walking, striding is less taxing on the lower-leg joints as the soles of an your shoes never leave the footpads. Striding is usually less intense than the StairMaster as the activity involves less of a vertical component, which requires you to lift the equivalent of your body mass.

The intensity of stationary cycling can vary widely. It can involve sprinting or intermittent increases in intensity with hill climbing, both of which will provide a greater stress to anaerobic systems, especially the lactic acid system. In addition to the intensity and duration, the timing of stationary cycling will affect blood sugar responses for any insulin user. Very intense cycling may actually cause blood sugar levels to rise, especially if you exercise in the morning.

"Skiing" indoors on the NordicTrack can bestow similar benefits as cross-country skiing if you use good technique, although most people do not use a NordicTrack for as long as they would go cross-country skiing outdoors, and they do not have to deal with a cold environment. As a result, this activity will generally have less of a glucose-lowering effect compared with the same outdoor activity.

The intensity and duration of rowing have the biggest effects on blood sugar control. Short, more intense rowing will maintain blood sugar more effectively due to a greater release of glucose-raising hormones during the activity. Longer, less intense rowing may require greater regimen changes to maintain blood sugar levels compared with outdoor rowing.

Athlete Examples

Insulin Changes Alone

For 35 minutes of StairMaster exercise after lunch, an NPH user usually decreases her prelunch Humalog by 15 percent and her bedtime NPH by 15 percent.

For NordicTrack exercise lasting for 25 to 30 minutes, an insulin pump user disconnects her pump. If her blood sugar is high to start, she may take a bolus (1 unit for every 50 mg/dl over normal) before disconnecting. She finds that she seldom has to eat any supplemental carbohydrate if she removes her insulin pump.

For exercise on a rowing machine, a pump user decreases his preexercise meal bolus by 30 to 35 percent. He maintains his normal basal rate during the activity, and he does not usually need to supplement with extra food.

Diet Changes Alone

A pump user finds that for every 20 to 30 minutes of stair climbing, she needs to eat an additional 30 grams of carbohydrates. She does not make any insulin adjustments unless she does the activity after a meal; then she reduces her premeal bolus slightly.

For 30 minutes of stationary cycling before breakfast, an NPH user does not make any insulin adjustments because he takes his insulin afterwards. He makes no dietary adjustments because he experiences no noticeable changes in his blood sugar level.

For 30 to 45 minutes on a stationary cycle, a pump user usually finds that she does not need to make any major adjustments in her food intake or insulin for this activity. Exercise too soon after dinner sometimes causes her to get hypoglycemic during and then hyperglycemic after cycling. Stationary cycling in the late evening (three to four hours after dinner) requires no immediate insulin or food changes as her blood sugars remain stable, but this activity tends to reduce her blood sugars during the night.

Combined Insulin and Diet Changes

For a postbreakfast workout on a StairMaster lasting 35 to 40 minutes at 80 percent intensity, an NPH user reduces her Humalog dose by 2 to 3 units if her fasting blood sugar is less than 100 mg/dl. Before exercise in the late afternoon, she eats 15 grams of carbohydrate if her blood sugar is less than 100 mg/dl, or nothing at all if it is more than 150.

An insulin pump user strides for 30 to 60 minutes at a time at a moderate pace. She disconnects her pump before exercising, and she finds that her blood sugar levels stay fairly constant during

AEROBIC CONDITIONING MACHINES

User	Insulin	Diet
NPH/Lente	• For shorter workouts of 20 minutes or less following a meal, reduce short-acting insulin doses by 0-20%. • For longer workouts lasting 30-60 minutes, reduce insulins by 20-40% depending on the time of day of the activity. • For workouts when circulating insulin levels are low, reduce insulin by 0-20% or increase carbohydrate. • You should not need to reduce bedtime NPH or Lente doses.	• For shorter workouts, increase carbohydrate intake by 5-15 grams. • For longer workouts, increase carbohydrates by 15-30 grams per hour depending on insulin reductions. • Make lesser carbohydrate increases at times when circulating insulin levels are lower.
Insulin Pump	• For shorter workouts of 20 minutes or less, reduce insulin boluses by 0-20%. • Reduce basal insulin rates by 25-50% during the activity, or remove the pump. • For longer workouts, reduce insulin boluses by 20-40% and/or reduce basal rate by 50-100% during exercise. • For workouts when circulating insulin levels are low, reduce basal rates alone or make no changes. • Maintain basal rate reductions of 25-50% following more prolonged exercise for 1-2 hours as well.	• For shorter workouts, increase carbohydrate intake by 5-15 grams for exercise. • For longer workouts, supplement with 15-25 grams of carbohydrate per hour. • Supplement with less carbohydrate when circulating insulin levels are lower during the activity.
Ultralente	• For shorter workouts of 20 minutes or less, reduce short-acting insulin doses by 0-20%. • For longer workouts, reduce insulin doses by 20-40% depending on the time of day of the activity. • For workouts when circulating insulin levels are low, make minimal changes in insulin. • Do not change Ultralente doses for these activities.	• For shorter workouts, increase carbohydrate intake by 5-25 grams. • For longer workouts, increase carbohydrate intake by 15 grams per hour. • Supplement with less carbohydrate (if any) when circulating insulin levels are lower.

the activity if her starting blood sugar is between 80 and 180 mg/dl. If her starting blood sugar is less than 80 mg/dl, she will supplement with 10 to 15 grams of carbohydrate, and if her blood sugar is over 180 mg/dl, she takes a bolus of 1 unit of Humalog before disconnecting.

Another NPH user rides an exercise bike at a moderate pace every evening for 60 minutes. She reduces her bedtime NPH dose by 0.5 to 2 units (she takes 8 to 8.5 units instead of 9 to 10), depending on her blood sugar reading at bedtime. She eats cookies or juice (15 grams of carbohydrate) before and after the activity as needed. She finds that her blood sugars drop more after the activity than during it.

An Ultralente user rides a stationary cycle at a moderate pace for 45 to 60 minutes at a time. She makes no alterations in her Ultralente dose, but she may reduce her premeal Regular by 1 unit if she does the activity within two hours after a meal. For late-afternoon or late-evening exercise, she makes no alterations, but supplements with carbohydrate if needed.

Intensity, Duration, and Other Effects

Effect of time of day. An NPH user makes no adjustments for a 15-minute StairMaster workout before dinner because the effects of her Humalog insulin are minimal at that time of day (she uses NPH at bedtime only). A pump user exercises for 40 minutes on the StairMaster in the early morning with high-speed intervals. She reduces her basal rate to 0.3 units per hour (from 0.5), and her blood sugar never gets low at that time of day.

Effect of time of day. For 30 to 60 minutes of stationary cycling before breakfast, an NPH user does not make any insulin adjustments because he takes his NPH and Humalog insulins after his exercise. He makes no dietary adjustments because he experiences no noticeable changes in his blood sugar level.

WALKING AND RACEWALKING

These activities are very aerobic in nature as they stress endurance. The body uses fats and carbohydrates as its main fuels. Carbohydrate use (both blood glucose and muscle glycogen) increases with walking intensity. Blood sugar responses will vary with the duration of walking as well as the intensity. No matter what regimen you follow, you can make alterations in insulin, diet, or a combination thereof, depending on other factors such as the time of day you walk, blood sugar levels, and circulating insulin levels during exercise.

NPH and Lente users. For NPH and Lente users, the biggest effect of walking appears to come from circulating insulin levels at the time of exercise. For moderate-paced walking early in the morning before your insulin injection, you may need no changes if your exercise lasts 60 minutes or less. If you exercise after a short-acting dose of insulin, the dose can be reduced. For planned exercise later in the day closer to an NPH peak, a 10 to 30 percent reduction in the morning NPH dose may be the most advantageous strategy. Longer, faster walks at any time of day (60 minutes or more at a 4-mph pace) will require greater changes in insulin and/or carbohydrate intakes.

Insulin pump users. Pump users have the most flexibility for walking as they can choose to suspend or reduce basal insulin rates during the activity, depending on the intensity and duration. A reduction in the basal rate provides the most normal physiological response to exercise by reducing the circulating levels of insulin. If the walking is slow to moderate in pace, a 25 percent reduction in the basal rate may suffice. For more intense or extended walks, you may need a 50 percent basal reduction as well as reduced boluses for snacks and meals during and following the activity.

Ultralente users. If you walk when circulating insulin levels are minimal (more than three to four hours after a meal), you may need fewer modifications than if you exercise closely following a meal when short-acting insulin levels are higher. You may not need any adjustments for slow or short walks soon after a meal. Longer or faster walks may still require some carbohydrate supplementation (15 to 30 grams per hour) due to exercise-stimulated glucose uptake by the muscles.

Athlete Examples

The following examples illustrate a variety of insulin and diet changes to compensate for everything from slow walking to racewalking to cross country walking.

Insulin Changes Alone

For walking 40 minutes at a 4-mph pace, an NPH user reduces his preexercise meal Humalog dose by 30 to 40 percent (4 units). To avoid hypoglycemia, he reduces his Humalog for the meal immediately following the activity by 25 percent (usually to 2 units) as well as his bedtime NPH by 25 percent.

WALKING AND RACEWALKING

User	Insulin	Diet
NPH/Lente	• For shorter or slower-paced walking, minimally reduce insulin doses (0-15%). • For longer or faster walking, reduce preexercise meal short-acting insulin by 20-40%. • For afternoon exercise (if NPH is taken in the morning), reduce your morning NPH dose by 10-30%. • Make fewer insulin changes if exercising with lower circulating insulin levels (before meals). • Consider reducing evening doses of NPH or Lente by 10-20% as well after a vigorous, prolonged walk.	• For slow-paced or short walks, make minimal increases in carbohydrates (0-10 grams) for the activity (and only if blood sugars are not hyperglycemic to start). • For longer or faster walking, increase carbohydrate intake by 10-20 grams prior to or during exercise. • For exercise done when circulating insulin levels are lower make no increase in carbohydrate intake.
Insulin Pump	• For slower or shorter walks, reduce basal insulin doses minimally (0-20%) during the activity. • For more extended efforts, reduce the basal rate during and/or boluses before exercise by 20-40%. • Walking while circulating insulin levels are lower (more than 3-4 hours following the last bolus of short-acting insulin) will require minimal insulin changes.	• For slow-paced or short walks, make minimal (if any) increases in carbohydrates (0-10 grams) for the activity, depending on starting blood sugar levels. • For longer, more intense walks, increase carbohydrate intake by 10-15 grams per hour, depending on insulin reductions.
Ultralente	• For slower, shorter walks, modify short-acting insulin by 0-20%. • Reduce short-acting insulin doses by 20-40% for meals before exercise to maintain blood sugar during longer, faster walking. • Make minimal insulin changes for walking while circulating insulin levels are lower (more than 3-4 hours after a dose of short-acting insulin or early in the morning). • Do not lower Ultralente doses for this activity unless walking is very prolonged.	• For shorter or slower walking make minimal increases in carbohydrate intake (0-10 grams), depending on starting blood sugar levels. • Increase carbohydrate intake by 10-15 grams per hour for longer, more intense walking to maintain blood sugar levels. • Make minimal increases in carbohydrate intake for walking when circulating insulin levels are minimal (more than 3-4 hours after the last injection of short-acting insulin).

For briskly walking 2.5 to 3 miles a day after breakfast, an insulin pump user decreases the basal rate on her pump to 0.1 units per hour for the duration of the exercise and keeps it down for 30 minutes after exercise. For a moderate walk, she may only decrease her basal rate by 0.2 to 0.4 units per hour (her usual is 0.6 to 0.8 units per hour) during the walk.

For racewalking for 60 to 90 minutes, another pump user disconnects her pump if her blood sugar is at least 110 mg/dl and less than 220. She needs to eat additional carbohydrate within an hour after finishing.

For mild walking for 30 to 35 minutes, an Ultralente user decreases her Humalog dose by 1 to 2 units (she usually takes 4 to 5 units) at the preceding meal. She also drinks extra juice if needed.

Diet Changes Alone

An NPH user race walks in the late afternoon. She usually eats more at lunch so that her blood sugar is around 200 mg/dl when she begins her walk. She does not eat an additional snack before walking, but she generally has low blood sugar when she finishes walking.

For walking seven to 14 miles in the morning, another NPH user usually eats one carbohydrate and one protein exchange before her walk, but she does not adjust her insulin. If she walks in the afternoon, she makes no adjustment in food or insulin.

A pump user does not adjust his basal rate if he walks less than 60 minutes, but he increases his carbohydrate consumption by 30 grams for every 30 minutes of walking without bolusing. For moderate walking for 20 to 60 minutes, another pump user does not usually alter the basal rate on her pump. She supplements with 15 grams of carbohydrate if needed. If she becomes hypoglycemic while walking, she reduces her basal rate by 50 percent for the remainder of the walk.

An Ultralente user walks 60 minutes a day. She does not adjust her insulin, but she eats extra food at the beginning of her walk if her blood sugar is below 130 mg/dl.

Combined Insulin and Diet Changes

For walking at 4 mph for more than 60 minutes, an NPH user reduces her breakfast Humalog by 2 to 3 units if her blood sugar is less than 100 mg/dl. For late-afternoon walks, she eats an additional 15 grams of carbohydrate if her blood sugar is less than 100 mg/dl. She eats nothing if it is more than 150 mg/dl. For long walks up to two hours, another NPH user decreases his short-acting insulins (a combination of Humalog and Regular) by 2 units at his preexercise meal. He also eats a snack after every four miles of walking.

For walking in the woods, a pump user reduces the basal rate on her pump by 50 percent (from 1.0 to 0.5 units per hour) 30 to 45 minutes before exercise. She also has a quick-acting carbohydrate such as a banana or four ounces of juice before her walk.

An Ultralente user decreases her Humalog by 1 unit before walking. She supplements with 15 grams of carbohydrate for every hour of the activity.

Intensity, Duration, and Other Effects

Effect of time of day. An NPH user walks early in the morning before her breakfast and morning dose of NPH and Humalog. She finds that she does not need any extra food due to the time of day and lack of insulin. She drinks some juice or eats a snack before walking later in the day. An Ultralente user finds that she can walk without any adjustments or additional food as long as her circulating insulin levels are minimal, at least three to four hours since her last injection of Humalog.

Effect of extended exercise. One pump user is a racewalker who usually walks 25 miles a day. He has participated in walks across the United States in the span of three summers. For this extended activity, he cuts his basal rate by almost 50 percent. He keeps his Humalog boluses the same but he eats more food. It works well for him to eat a slow-acting energy bar twice a day while walking all day. He also ingests 10 to 20 grams of carbohydrate every hour and tests his blood sugar frequently.

WEIGHT AND RESISTANCE CIRCUIT TRAINING

Weight training involves short, powerful repetitions of a specific movement that utilize mainly anaerobic energy sources (stored phosphagens and muscle glycogen via the lactic acid system). Circuit training usually emphasizes a greater number of repetitions with lower resistance and is slightly more aerobic in nature, although still primarily anaerobic. You may need minimal changes in insulin or diet to maintain blood sugar levels due to the intense nature of this activity. However, a prolonged weight-training session powerlifting may result in significant glycogen depletion, thus increasing your risk of later-onset hypoglycemia.

The intensity of weight training affects blood sugar levels. The time of day you exercise and circulating insulin levels at the time also affect blood sugar maintenance. The intensity of individual weightlifting sets affects the release of glucose-raising hormones. As a result, many people may find that they can maintain blood sugar levels during this activity with few changes in their diabetic regimen. Blood sugars will be even more stable, or perhaps rise, during weight training at times when circulating insulin levels are lower (more than three to four hours since the last injection of short-acting insulin) or early in the morning when insulin resistance is higher. At these times, you may actually need supplemental insulin to counter the resultant rise in blood sugar levels. However, a prolonged weight-training session may result in significant glycogen depletion that may increase risk for later-onset hypoglycemia.

Many people often do weight training in combination with an aerobic workout on a stationary cycle, rowing machine, StairMaster, treadmill, or other type of exercise equipment. In these cases, you may need greater regimen changes but not as many changes as aerobic exercise alone would require due to the effects of the weight training. You will need to monitor blood sugars closely later in the day following a weight-training session and you can make corrections in insulin or diet then to prevent later-onset hypoglycemia.

Athlete Examples

The following examples illustrate the variety of regimen changes required for weight training. The intensity, duration, and the time of day of weight training all have different effects on blood sugar.

Insulin Changes Alone

For training at home with free weights and a weight machine after dinner, an NPH user reduces her predinner Humalog by 2 units. For weight training three hours in the morning, another NPH user reduces his prebreakfast Humalog by about 1 unit, but he does not make any changes in his breakfast intake. For one to

WEIGHT AND RESISTANCE CIRCUIT TRAINING

User	Insulin	Diet
NPH/Lente	• Either no change, minimal reductions, or minimal increases in insulin may be necessary to maintain blood sugar levels during weight training, depending on timing, intensity, and duration. • For weight training after a meal, prolonged training of 2 hours or more, or training combined with an aerobic workout, reduce short-acting insulin by 10-20%. • For weight training more than 3-4 hours after the last injection of short-acting insulin, either make no regimen change or take a small dose of supplemental insulin (1-2 units) afterward to correct increased blood sugar levels.	• Increase carbohydrate intake by 0-20 grams per hour depending on exercise intensity and duration.
Insulin Pump	• Maintain normal basal rates during this activity or disconnect insulin pump depending on the intensity and duration of lifting. • When weightlifting without doing any conditioning workout, maintain insulin basal rates to prevent increases in blood sugars. • When training in combination with an aerobic workout, disconnect the pump during both activities to maintain blood sugars. • When weightlifting immediately following a meal, reduce the premeal bolus by 10-20%.	• For prolonged training sessions of 2 hours or more, consume 0-20 grams of supplemental carbohydrates per hour.
Ultralente	• Make minimal alterations in short-acting insulins to maintain blood sugar levels during this activity. • For weight training closely following a meal, prolonged training of 2 hours or more, or training combined with an aerobic workout, reduce short-acting insulin by 10-20%. • For weight training more than 3-4 hours after the last injection of short-acting insulin, either make no change or take a small dose of supplemental insulin (1-2 units) after the activity if needed to correct increased blood sugar levels. • Do not alter Ultralente doses for weight training.	• For prolonged training, consider an increase in carbohydrate intake of 0-20 grams per hour depending on exercise intensity.

two hours of training later in the day, another NPH user reduces her morning NPH dose by 1 unit (from 6 to 5 units) and snacks before and after the activity if her blood sugar is low.

A pump user turns off his insulin pump during his circuit training workouts but does not significantly modify his food intake. For weight training alone, another pump user does not adjust his basal rate. When combining weight training with a general cardiovascular workout on aerobic conditioning machines, he will often reduce his basal rate by 50 percent for three hours during his training and supplement with a sport drink.

Another pump user usually does 20 to 25 minutes of weight training after 30 to 45 minutes of StairMaster or running. She disconnects her pump for the aerobic portion and she leaves it disconnected during the weight training. She makes no dietary adjustments for these activities before lunch.

For moderate weight training, another pump user does not adjust her basal rate or her boluses before the workout, but she finds that her blood sugars drop about four hours later, so she may reduce her next meal bolus or her basal rate.

Another Ultralente user makes sure that he does not take any Humalog within two hours of weight training unless his blood sugar is 180 mg/dl or above, and he eats a snack before weightlifting if his blood sugar is less than 100 mg/dl.

Diet Changes Alone

An NPH user does not adjust his insulin for weight training, but he eats a higher-fat bedtime snack on the days that he does this activity to prevent nocturnal hypoglycemia.

Another NPH user usually does weight training for 90 minutes and only eats 15 grams of carbohydrate if his blood sugar is 85 mg/dl or less to start. Otherwise, he makes no dietary or insulin changes for his workout.

A pump user finds that he needs to make no changes in his basal rate during weight training. He eats about 45 grams of carbohydrate before his workout and checks his blood sugar after 60 minutes of training.

An Ultralente user does weight training for 45 minutes following either running or aerobics. She does not take any insulin for this activity, and she usually has a sport drink during the activity because her blood sugars tend to drop.

Combined Insulin and Diet Changes

For a combined 90-minute workout with weights and the stationary cycle, an NPH user decreases his preexercise Humalog by 1 unit. After his workouts, he finds that he needs to take only 1 unit of Humalog per 30 grams of carbohydrate instead of his usual dose of 1 unit per 20 grams.

An Ultralente user participates in bodybuilding contests that require him to weight train at least three days a week for 30 to 60 minutes. He waits until he finishes exercising to inject any Humalog, and he adjusts his dose to match his carbohydrate consumption, which is relatively low. Another Ultralente user makes no adjustments to his insulin or diet for one to two hours of moderate weight training.

Intensity, Duration, and Other Effects

Effect of intensity. An NPH user finds that weight training does not require any modifications, but sometimes it will trigger a slight drop in his blood sugar several hours later. For intense weight training, a pump user makes no adjustments in her insulin or food intake if her starting blood sugar is between 145 and 180 mg/dl. Another pump user finds that doing a 40-minute weight-training circuit after dinner can actually cause his blood sugar to rise by the end of the session. He often has to bolus an additional 0.5 units to cover the increase in his blood sugar.

A pump user finds that if she does weight training alone, it often causes her blood sugar levels to increase, but in combination with a regular cardiovascular workout, she makes no adjustments. An Ultralente user finds that lifting weights tends to increase his blood sugars so he tries to prevent this with cross-training. His weightlifting consists of interspersing five to 10 minutes of aerobic exercise on the NordicTrack, treadmill, or stationary bike between each weightlifting activity.

Effect of time of day. An NPH user does weight training for 45 minutes before dinner. She makes no adjustments in insulin or diet. Another NPH user makes no dietary or insulin adjustments for weight training before lunch. He eats his usual midmorning snack and then weight trains for 60 minutes with no significant drop in his blood sugars. For 75-minute workouts with weights, another NPH user does not make any insulin adjustments or changes in his diet because he exercises in the morning before breakfast and his insulin injection of NPH and Humalog. An Ultralente user finds that her blood sugars stay quite stable during circuit training as long as it has been three to four hours since her last injection of Humalog.

MARTIAL ARTS

These activities include karate, judo, taekwondo, and t'ai chi, and are both anaerobic and aerobic in nature, depending on the intensity of the activity. Most involve power moves like kicking or chopping, and some disciplines, such as t'ai chi, include slow, controlled movements that are more prolonged and less intense aerobic moves. The intensity and duration of the workout determine the necessary regimen changes.

The intensity of any martial arts activity will have the main effect on blood glucose levels. Very intense workouts will be more anaerobic in nature and may not cause much of a decrease in blood sugar levels during the activity. In some cases, martial arts can cause blood sugars to increase due to the intense nature and the release of glucose-raising hormones. You should anticipate delayed decreases in blood sugar levels following prolonged, intense workouts that cause significant depletion of muscle glycogen. A less intense activity such as t'ai chi may require minimal regimen changes because of its low-level aerobic nature.

Athlete Examples

These examples demonstrate the need to modify each regimen according to the type, intensity, duration, and timing of martial arts workouts.

MARTIAL ARTS

User	Insulin	Diet
NPH/Lente	• Reduce short-acting insulin doses by 0-30% before doing martial arts, depending on the type, intensity, and duration of training. • Lower morning NPH or lente doses (if taken) a similar amount for afternoon participation. • Make greater insulin reductions for more vigorous activities such as judo or karate compared with lower-activity martial arts such as t'ai chi. • Consider giving a supplemental dose of short-acting insulin (1-2 units) following intense martial arts competitions if blood sugar have risen.	• Supplement with 0-15 grams of carbohydrate per hour depending on the intensity of the activity. • For higher-intensity workouts or martial arts competitions, you should not need extra carbohydrate. Watch for later-onset hypoglycemia.
Insulin Pump	• Reduce basal insulin rates by 0-30% during the activity. • For longer workouts (1-2 hours), reduce insulin boluses before the workout by 10-25%. • More vigorous activities such as judo or karate may require greater reductions than lower-activity martial arts such as t'ai chi. • Consider giving a supplemental bolus of short-acting insulin (1-2 units) following intense martial arts competitions if blood sugar have risen.	• Supplement with 0-15 grams of carbohydrate per hour as needed for blood sugar maintenance. • For higher-intensity workouts or martial arts competitions, you should not need to consume extra carbohydrate during the activity.
Ultralente	• Reduce short-acting insulin doses preexercise by 0-30% for the activity. • For longer workouts (1-2 hours), reduce insulin doses before the workout by 10-25%. • Make greater changes for more vigorous activities such as judo or karate compared with lower-activity martial arts such as t'ai chi. • Consider giving a supplemental dose of short-acting insulin (1-2 units) following intense martial arts competitions if blood sugars have risen. • Do not make changes in Ultralente doses for weight training.	• Supplement with 0-15 grams of carbohydrate per hour as needed for blood sugar maintenance. • For higher-intensity workouts or martial arts competitions, you should not need extra carbohydrate during the activity.

Insulin Changes Alone

For 60 minutes of intense karate, an NPH user eats half of his usual dinner before the workout, but he only takes a third of his usual Humalog to cover his food (4 units instead of 12). Sometimes he decreases his bedtime NPH to prevent nocturnal hypoglycemia.

Diet Changes Alone

For taekwondo, a bedtime-only NPH user eats hard candy before 60-minute workouts. She does not adjust her insulin dose. Another NPH user and a pump user increase their food intake before 60- to 90-minute sessions of karate but they do not adjust their insulin doses.

Combined Insulin and Diet Changes

For karate sessions lasting one to two hours, an NPH user eliminates his Humalog dose before meals (3 to 5 units) and eats additional carbohydrate before and during the exercise based on his blood glucose levels.

For taekwondo, a pump user reduces his predinner Humalog bolus by 3 units but does not adjust the basal rate on his pump. He drinks six to eight ounces of orange juice if his blood sugar gets too low during the activity.

Intensity, Duration, and Other Effects

Effect of intensity. For 60 minutes of high-intensity taekwondo, an Ultralente user makes no adjustments to his insulin or diet. His blood sugars remain stable during this activity.

BOXING

This activity involves short, powerful jabs and quick movements (anaerobic) as well as more constant movement of the legs during a given round. Training for boxing is usually a combination of power and endurance movements. For possible regimen changes, refer to recommendations for kickboxing in the next section.

Athlete Examples

For a 60-minute workout video of regular boxing, an NPH user does not change her insulin, but she tests her blood sugar and snacks if necessary before starting. An Ultralente user makes few regimen adjustments because she "boxercises" with little circulating insulin (no recent Humalog injections); otherwise, she finds that it can cause rapid drops in her blood sugars.

KICKBOXING

Kickboxing is mostly anaerobic, involving short bursts of powerful movements. It may also involve more continual movement of the legs during a given round. Training for kickboxing is usually a combination of power and endurance movements designed to increase muscular strength as well as muscular endurance. Regimen changes will depend on the intensity and duration of this activity as well as the time of day you exercise.

The intensity of boxing and the circulating insulin levels during a workout or competition have the biggest effects on blood sugar levels. A higher-intensity, more anaerobic workout will often require few regimen changes due to the greater release of glucose-raising hormones. In this case, if your starting blood sugar levels are higher than normal, the exercise can actually cause those levels to increase, requiring an additional dose of short-acting insulin. If you have a low amount of circulating insulin levels during such a high-intensity activity, then you will need even fewer regimen changes for blood sugar maintenance.

Athlete Examples

These examples show that varied changes work well for different people.

Insulin Changes Alone

For aerobic kickboxing classes, an NPH user alters her regimen according to her starting blood sugar. If her blood sugar is around 120 mg/dl, she makes no dietary or insulin changes; if higher, she may take a small dose of Humalog before class.

KICKBOXING

User	Insulin	Diet
NPH/Lente	• Reduce short-acting insulin by 10-30% depending on expected intensity and duration of training. • For afternoon workouts, reduce morning doses of NPH or Lente (if taken) by 10-25%. • For longer workouts (1-3 hours), reduce short-acting insulin prior to the workout by 20-30%. • For high-intensity workouts or those done when circulating insulin levels are lower make lesser reductions in insulin, and possibly supplement with a dose of short-acting insulin (1-2 units) if starting blood sugars are above normal.	• Depending on the workout intensity, increase carbohydrate intake by 5-15 grams per hour. • Make minimal carbohydrate increases for shorter, less intense workouts. • Supplement with 15 grams of carbohydrates or more per hour for longer duration (1-3 hours) workouts, depending on insulin changes. • If exercise is done when circulating levels of insulin are low (more than 3-4 hours after the last short-acting insulin dose), make minimal increases in carbohydrate intake.
Insulin Pump	• Reduce short-acting boluses of insulin preexercise by 10-30% depending on intensity and duration of training. • Lower insulin basal rates by 10-40% alone or along with bolus decreases. • For higher-intensity workouts, consider bolusing with 1-2 units of supplemental insulin to counter above-normal starting blood sugars. • For longer workouts (1-3 hours), make greater reductions in insulin prior to or during the workout. • Make lesser insulin changes to compensate for exercise done when circulating insulin levels are lower (early morning or more than 3-4 hours since the last insulin bolus).	• Depending on intensity of workout, increase carbohydrate intake by 5-15 grams per hour. • Make lesser carbohydrate changes for shorter, less intense workouts. • Supplement with 10-15 grams or more carbohydrate per hour for longer duration workouts (1-3 hours), depending on insulin reductions. • If exercising when circulating levels of insulin are low, make minimal increases in carbohydrate intake.
Ultralente	• Reduce short-acting insulin by 10-30% depending on intensity and duration of training. • For higher-intensity workouts, consider supplementing with a small dose of short-acting insulin (1-2 units) before exercise for elevated starting blood sugars. • For longer workouts (1-3 hours), reduce short-acting insulin prior to the workout. • Make minimal insulin reductions for exercise done when circulating insulin levels are lower.	• Depending on intensity of workout, increase carbohydrates by 5-15 grams per hour. • Make lesser increases for shorter, less intense workouts. • For longer duration workouts (1-3 hours), supplement with 10-15 grams of carbohydrate or more per hour, depending on circulating insulin levels and exercise intensity. • If exercise is done when insulin levels are lower, increase carbohydrate intake minimally.

Diet Changes Alone

For 60 minutes of cardio kickboxing, an NPH user does not adjust his insulin, but he does drink some orange juice and a sweetened ice tea before the workout. A pump user eats additional carbohydrate before his workout but does not adjust his insulin doses.

Combined Insulin and Diet Changes

In training for kickboxing competitions, an NPH user reduces his morning NPH by 2 units and his lunch Humalog by 3 units before the afternoon training session. He also eats more simple sugars before the workout. Another NPH user decreases his dinner dose of NPH by 2 units and his predinner Humalog by 3 units before kickboxing training for one to three hours in the evenings. He also eats more simple sugars and monitors his blood sugar after workouts.

Intensity, Duration, and Other Effects

Effect of circulating insulin levels. For a 75-minute class before dinner, an NPH user eats a snack before beginning based on her blood sugars: If her blood sugar is around 80 mg/dl, she eats 30 grams of carbohydrate, but she eats only 15 grams if her blood sugar is 130 mg/dl. On her workout days, she takes no Humalog in the afternoon, so hypoglycemia is infrequent due to her low circulating insulin levels at the time of the class. Another NPH user leads 70-minute high-intensity kickboxing classes. She will sometimes take an additional 1 to 2 units of Humalog because her blood sugars tend to run higher in the late afternoon. If her blood sugar is less than 200 mg/dl, she will not usually take any insulin. If it is more than 200, she takes 1 to 2 units before the class.

YOGA AND STRETCHING

These activities are very low-level in nature and require minimal muscular effort. Most stretches, especially in yoga, are static (involving no movement) and are held for a period of time. Thus, minimal energy is used. Joint and muscle flexibility are often limited by long-term diabetes and can be improved through these activities. You should need neither dietary nor insulin changes regardless of your insulin regimen. Even yoga classes lasting for an hour or more will use minimal amounts of energy.

Fitness activities run the gamut from extremely low level activities like yoga to vigorous activities such as aerobic dance or weight training. Your blood sugar responses to these varying activities can be effectively managed to allow you to participate in any and all of them.

Chapter 10

Recreational Sports

Have you ever dreamed of walking across the United States, backpacking in the Sierra Nevada mountains, diving in the Caribbean Sea, or white-water canoeing down a dangerous river? Maybe you have watched the Winter Olympics and seen athletes skiing down mountains at incredible speeds and wished you could do that too, or maybe the slower pace and scenery of cross-country skiing is more your speed. In any case, people with diabetes have done all of these activities and many more while maintaining control over their blood sugar levels.

This chapter gives recommendations for regimen changes and real-life examples of the following recreational physical activities: hiking and backpacking, rock climbing, mountain biking, horseback riding, skydiving, canoeing and kayaking, windsurfing, surfing and boogieboarding, scuba diving, snorkeling, waterskiing, jetskiing, snowmobiling, sailing, beach volleyball, downhill skiing and snowboarding, snowshoeing, ice and in-line skating, skateboarding, golf, tennis, indoor racket sports (racquetball, handball, squash, and badminton), dance (ballet, modern, social, and ballroom), bowling, yardwork, and exercise under environmental extremes.

These recreational sports and activities vary widely in their use of the body's fuels. Some activities are intense and brief, such as a golf swing, and are primarily fueled by the phosphagens (ATP and CP) stored in muscles. Others involve the lactic acid system (glycolysis) as well due to their intense but more prolonged nature (for example, rock climbing). Many of these activities rely primarily on aerobic sources of energy such as carbohydrate and fat, especially prolonged activities such as backpacking. These activities intermittently rely on anaerobic energy sources to cover brief increases in intensity. Chapter 2 fully discusses the various energy systems and energy sources used for different types of exercise.

Giving any overall general recommendations for regimen changes for all recreational activities is problematic as they are so varied and run the gamut from extremely low-level activities such as bowling to intense, prolonged activities such as backpacking or mountain biking. The intensity and duration of some of these activities vary greatly even within the activity itself (e.g., downhill skiing). As a result, no overall recommendations can be given for these activities as a whole.

For each sport or activity, however, general recommendations as well as real-life examples of some athlete's specific changes in insulin and diet are listed according to their insulin regimen (NPH and Lente, insulin pump, and Ultralente users). *If you only use oral hypoglycemic agents, this regimen is not listed separately, but you can use the general recommendations under diet changes for NPH and Lente users as an approximate guide when your blood sugars at the start of or during*

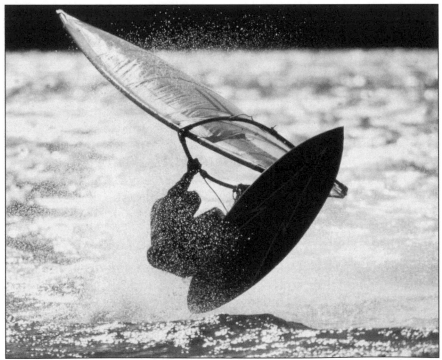

© Kevin Vandivier

Windsurfing can be an intense recreational activity that requires you to make substantial regimen changes.

exercise are in a normal range. When your blood sugars are elevated, you will need to make few, if any, dietary increases for exercise. Your risk for hypoglycemia may be higher depending on the type of medication that you use. You should consult a physician before making any reductions in oral medication doses to compensate for these activities. Refer to chapter 3 for more information about the actions of various types of insulins and oral hypoglycemic agents.

GENERAL RECOMMENDATIONS

Overall recommendations are given for changes in insulin and diet that generally apply to all diabetic medication regimens (insulin and oral agents). Refer to each activity for more sport-specific recommendations.

Combined Insulin and Diet Changes

For either short or low-intensity activities such as recreational ice skating, you will usually need no reductions in insulin doses or increases in carbohydrate intake. For more intense activities such as beach volleyball, some limited extra carbohydrate intake will be appropriate alone or in combination with reduced insulin doses, depending on how long you do the activity. For prolonged activities such as snowshoeing, you will need increases in carbohydrate intake along with reduced insulin doses to maintain blood sugar levels during and following the activity.

Intensity, Duration, and Other Effects

This wide array of recreational activities will elicit many different blood sugar responses depending on intensity, duration, and environmental conditions, among other factors. Low-intensity activities such as snorkeling or bowling may have minimal impact on blood sugars. More intense and prolonged activities such as tennis, racquetball, or rock climbing may require much greater insulin and food changes to maintain blood sugar levels. The effects of heat, cold, or altitude conditions can be sizeable also, causing a greater than normal use of stored muscle glycogen and blood glucose (carbohydrates) that you would need to counter with regimen changes.

HIKING AND BACKPACKING

Both hiking and backpacking are very aerobic in nature because they stress the walking endurance to cover longer distances more slowly, and they are often done carrying extra weight, especially in the case of backpacking. The body's main fuels are fat and carbohydrate, and both are important in such prolonged activities. More carbohydrate (blood glucose and muscle glycogen) are used with any increase in intensity. For hiking, you can alter either insulin doses or food intake or both, depending on your desire for additional food during the activity, but you will usually need changes in both insulin and diet for backpacking due to its prolonged nature. The length of time you spend doing these activities (hours or days), the extra weight you carry, and the environmental conditions can all have an impact on blood sugar response and the necessary regimen changes.

Environmental conditions such as altitude, cold, and heat and humidity affect hikers and backpackers. All of these conditions will decrease insulin requirements because they increase the body's energy expenditure. Altitude and cold, especially, will increase blood glucose utilization; under those conditions, the risk of hypoglycemia is higher. Hot and humid conditions can predispose hikers to dehydration (mainly through increased sweating), and so you should be especially careful to drink plenty of fluids. The body also uses more energy when trying to cool itself, thus increasing the risk for hypoglycemia.

The terrain you cover can also have an effect on blood sugar. Uphill climbing will require more energy than the downhill portions. Also, extremely strenuous uphill sections may actually cause a temporary rise in blood sugar levels due to an exaggerated release of glucose-raising hormones, especially when circulating insulin levels are low. Insulin requirements may actually increase, albeit temporarily, under these conditions. The risk for later occurrences of hypoglycemia (especially at night) following such a strenuous activity is a more important concern, and you will probably need to decrease insulin levels during the night to prevent nocturnal hypoglycemia.

Athlete Examples

These examples show the extreme changes in diet and insulin for hiking and backpacking, especially under more extreme environ-

HIKING

User	Insulin	Diet
NPH/Lente	• For shorter hikes up to 3 hours, decrease preexercise meal short-acting insulin by 10-30%. • For longer hikes of 4-6 hours, reduce the morning dose of NPH or Lente by 15-40% in addition to the reductions in the short-acting doses. • In addition, reduce bedtime NPH or Lente doses by 10-30% to prevent nocturnal hypoglycemia following the activity, especially if the exercise is unusual or prolonged.	• Eat additional snacks (10-25 grams) as dictated by blood sugars during a short hike. • Consume 10-30 grams of carbohydrate per hour of hiking in addition to the reductions in insulin for longer hikes.
Insulin Pump	• For shorter hikes of no more than 3 hours, reduce basal insulin rates by 25-50% as needed according to blood sugar levels. • Reduce preexercise meal bolus by 10-30%. • For longer hikes of 5-6 hours or more, reduce the basal insulin dose by 50-75%. • It is also possible to maintain basal levels and just eat snacks while hiking without taking a bolus dose. • Following exceptionally strenuous hiking or constant snacking, blood sugars can actually rise following the activity. Blood sugar monitoring determines the need for an additional bolus after cessation of all activity. • Reduce overnight basal rates by 10-25% to prevent nocturnal hypoglycemia, especially for unusual exercise or multiple-day hiking trips.	• Increase carbohydrate intake by 10-25 grams for short hikes. • Consume carbohydrate with either no additional insulin or a reduced bolus only if blood sugars begin to rise for longer hikes.
Ultralente	• For shorter hikes of 1-3 hours, reduce short-acting insulin doses by 10-30%. • For longer hikes of 5-6 hours or more, it may be necessary to reduce short-acting insulin for meals by 25-50%. • Following exceptionally strenuous hiking or constant snacking, blood sugars can actually rise following the activity. Blood sugar monitoring determines the need for additional short-acting insulin after cessation of all hiking for the day. • Reduce overnight Ultralente doses by 10-25% to prevent nocturnal hypoglycemia, especially for unusual exercise or multiple-day hiking trips.	• For shorter hikes, consider an increase in carbohydrate intake of 10-25 grams per hour during the hike. • For longer hikes, eat additional carbohydrate snacks with no additional insulin unless blood sugars increase.

BACKPACKING*

User	Insulin	Diet
NPH/Lente	• For multiple-day backpacking trips, reduce both intermediate- and short-acting insulin doses. • Reduce morning doses of NPH or Lente by 30-60%, and reduce short-acting doses by 25-50%. • Monitor blood sugar during the night until you correctly reduce the bedtime NPH dose by 10-40%.	• Eat a bedtime snack containing 15-30 grams of carbohydrate and possibly extra protein and fat. • In addition, increase food intake by 50% while backpacking even with the reductions in insulin.
Insulin Pump	• Reduce the basal rate by 50% during the activity as needed to maintain normal blood sugar levels (10-30 grams per hour or more if basal insulin is not reduced). • Decrease insulin doses by 25-50% for meals during and following the activity. • Reduce basal rates at night by 10-30%.	• Eat an extra snack of 15-30 grams of carbohydrate plus extra protein and fat before bedtime. • Eat additional carbohydrate without bolusing during the activity.
Ultralente	• Reduce Ultralente doses by as much as 50% before the activity. • Reduce insulin by 25-50% for meals during and following the activity. • Reduce meal boluses further if you do not significantly alter Ultralente doses. • Reduce overnight Ultralente doses by 10-30% following the activity.	• Eat an extra snack of 15-30 grams of carbohydrate with extra protein and fat before bedtime. • Eat additional carbohydrate without bolusing during the activity.

* For backpacking, a combination of less insulin and more food is usually necessary to compensate for the prolonged, strenuous nature of this activity. Several days of backpacking may have a cumulative effect on blood sugars, resulting in an increasing risk for nocturnal hypoglycemia as muscle glycogen levels may not be fully restored.

mental conditions. Backpackers cannot make diet changes alone to compensate although hikers often can.

Insulin Changes Alone for Hiking

An NPH user significantly reduces her Humalog for meals throughout the day (by 2 to 4 units depending on glucose readings) for all-day hikes. She may also reduce her bedtime NPH by 20 percent following the activity.

While hiking, an Ultralente user takes 0 to 50 percent of his usual Humalog for meals. If he hikes for more than one day, he decreases his Ultralente doses by 25 percent as well.

Diet Changes Alone for Hiking

When hiking, an NPH user snacks with a greater frequency than usual on foods like trail mix without adjusting her insulin dose.

For two-hour hikes, a pump user checks her blood sugar before beginning and tries to be between 145 and 180 mg/dl. If her blood sugars are lower, she eats half a Z-Bar or PowerBar and checks her blood sugars hourly.

Combined Insulin and Diet Changes for Hiking

For hiking five to six hours along a rocky, mountainous coastline, an NPH user decreases his morning Humalog by 4 to 5 units, his lunch dose by 0 to 4 units, his dinner dose by 2 to 4 units, and his bedtime snack dose by 2 to 3 units (down to 0) while maintaining his NPH doses, which consist of a large dose at bedtime and a small dose in the morning. He monitors his blood sugars every hour, eats lots of snacks, and keeps hydrated with sport drinks and soda.

A pump user reduces her Humalog bolus before meals by 2 units and also temporarily decreases her basal rate by 80 percent (0.5 unit per hour reduced to 0.1 unit) while hiking for three to four hours. She also supplements with orange juice or raisins as needed. On the third day of hiking during a recent hiking trip, she additionally reduced her basal rate by 0.1 unit per hour for a period of 48 hours.

For hiking over rugged terrain, another pump user decreases her bolus rate to 0.1 unit per hour (from 0.3 or 0.2 unit). She snacks at least hourly on the uphill portions without insulin. Her lunch bolus while hiking is a normal dose to counteract all the snacking with reduced boluses and her reduced basal rate. She takes insulin with snacks on the downhill portions. She often finds that her blood sugar begins to rise after she stops hiking, and she may need an additional bolus of insulin then.

Combined Insulin and Diet Changes for Backpacking

For backpacking two to three days, an NPH user allows himself a little less rigid glucose control than normal. He increases his food intake, drinks a diluted sport drink all day while hiking, and always has a bedtime snack. For trips of three to 10 days, he cuts back on his NPH by about 40 percent and reduces his Humalog by 25 to 50 percent for meals during the day.

For multiday backpacking trips in the mountains, a pump user finds the first 90 minutes to be critical. She reduces the basal rate on her pump by 50 percent (from 1.0 to 0.5 unit per hour) 30 to 45 minutes before the exercise begins. At the start, she also eats a quick-acting carbohydrate such as a banana. If she can stabilize her blood sugar in that time, then she keeps her basal rate reduced to 0.7 unit per hour and eats a small meal without a Humalog bolus. She reduces her basal rate at night by 0.1 unit per hour and eats a larger snack before bedtime.

For longer hikes of 20 miles or backpacking, an Ultralente user reduces her dose the night before as well as the morning of the activity by 50 percent. She eats 20 grams of carbohydrate just before beginning without taking any Humalog. During the hike she drinks diluted sport drinks and carries glucose tablets with her. She eats small quantities of carbohydrates after the activity and doses with Humalog according to her blood sugar readings. She resumes her normal Ultralente doses after stopping.

For mountaineering hikes of one day to one week, another Ultralente user decreases his total insulin by at least by 50 percent. Sometimes he does not take any Ultralente insulin at all and instead uses multiple small injections of Regular along the trail (even though he usually uses Humalog) along with frequent snacks along the trail.

Intensity, Duration, and Other Effects of Hiking

Effect of exercise intensity. A pump user hikes the Grand Canyon rim to rim every year (22.3 miles). For this activity, he decreases his basal rate by 50 percent, triples his carbohydrate intake, decreases his boluses by 50 percent (using an insulin-to-carbohydrate ratio of 1:20 instead of his usual 1:10). At the conclusion of the 13-mile uphill portion, he boluses 5 units of Humalog to cover the surge in his blood sugar at the end of his hike.

Effect of multiple days of strenuous activity. For all-day mountaineering, a pump user decreases her basal rate by 0.2 unit an hour while exercising. She tries to start hiking with her blood sugar above 150 mg/dl. She checks it after 30 minutes of the activity: If it drops below 100, she drinks eight ounces of a sport drink. She eats more snacks during the day (bagels, M&M's) and monitors her blood sugar in an attempt to keep it in the 100 to 150 mg/dl range. For subsequent days of mountaineering, she finds that she needs to decrease her basal rates by 0.1 to 0.3 unit per hour all the time.

Effect of heat and humidity. For hiking during the summer, an NPH user either decreases her insulin by 30 to 40 percent or she consumes 15 grams of carbohydrate per hour if hiking at a higher intensity and in the sun with increased humidity.

Effect of altitude. An Ultralente user decreases her Humalog insulin by up to 75 percent while hiking at altitude in the Swiss Alps and constantly consumes Swiss chocolate (one large block every two hours), dried fruits, bananas, apples, and sport drinks. She also finds that at altitude, she generally has to take twice her usual amount of quick-acting carbohydrate during the exercise.

Intensity, Duration, and Other Effects of Backpacking

Effect of intensity. A pump user takes backpacking trips for one to seven days. When she hikes up to 20 miles a day while carrying a backpack at higher altitudes, she reduces her basal rate to 0.2 units per hour from 0.5. She adjusts her insulin-to-carbohydrate ratio from 1:14 to 1 unit of Humalog for 30 to 45 grams of carbohydrate. If hiking hard uphill, she reduces her basal rate even further to 0.1 units per hour.

Effect of heat and humidity. For a day of backpacking in the Shenandoah mountains, an NPH user decreases his Humalog during the day by 20 to 30 percent before, during, and after the activity. During summer hikes, he supplements with cool sport drinks of less than 9 percent glucose. He also eats additional carbohydrate in his meal before starting as well as for three hours following cessation of activity to prevent postexercise hypoglycemia.

Effect of altitude. On a backpacking trip that she hiked for six to eight hours a day at altitude for three weeks, an NPH user decreased her total insulin intake by 60 percent (with reductions of both short-acting insulin during the day and bedtime NPH) and doubled her usual food intake.

Effect of cold temperatures. An NPH user does backpacking trips of two to five days. She finds that sleeping in a tent, especially in the cold, requires less insulin than sleeping at home, so the first night of her trip she reduces her NPH dose by 30 percent. During the day while hiking with her backpack, she usually reduces all Humalog doses by 20 to 30 percent. She usually increases her carbohydrate intake by 50 percent, mostly through snacking.

ROCK CLIMBING

This activity is a combination of anaerobic and aerobic movements. Because it is continuous over a period of time, it is somewhat aerobic, but a lot of the movements are quick and intense (grabbing and pulling) with rest periods in between moves, making it more of a strength-related activity. Changes in insulin or diet will depend on the intensity and duration of rock climbing activities.

Both the intensity of climbing and the duration will have an effect on the blood sugar response. More intense climbing may initially maintain blood sugars (due to a greater hormonal release) but results in greater muscle glycogen depletion and greater risk for later-onset hypoglycemia. Prolonged climbing will increase muscle glycogen use as well and require greater regimen changes. The more intense the climbing is and the longer it lasts, the greater the risk for hypoglycemia during the later stages and following the activity.

Athlete Examples

These real-life regimen changes show that you can use changes in insulin, diet, or usually both to compensate for this activity. The regimen adjustments differ when you rock climb for longer periods or more intensely.

Insulin Changes Alone

An NPH user eats a normal diet for this activity but decreases his regular insulin by 20 percent and his NPH dose by 50 percent

ROCK CLIMBING

User	Insulin	Diet
NPH/Lente	• Reduce short-acting insulin 25-50% before climbing to maintain blood sugar levels. • For more intense, all-day climbing, reduce morning doses of NPH (if taken) by 10-30%.	• Increase carbohydrate intake up to 15 grams before climbing. • Eat 10-30 grams of additional carbohydrate per hour if the activity is intense and prolonged.
Insulin Pump	• Reduce short-acting insulin by 25-50% before climbing. • Reduce basal insulin rates by 0-50% during short, active climbing. • For all-day climbing, reduce basal rates by slightly more (10-60%) during the activity.	• Consume up to15 grams of carbohydrate before climbing to maintain blood sugar levels. • Eat up to 30 grams of additional carbohydrate per hour for a longer activity depending on reductions in basal insulin rates.
Ultralente	• Reduce short-acting insulin by 25-50% before climbing. • For all-day climbing, reduce morning doses of Ultralente by 10-20%.	• Consume up to 15 grams of carbohydrate before climbing to maintain blood sugar levels. • Eat 10-30 grams of additional carbohydrate per hour for climbing all day.

before climbing. An Ultralente user decreases his preexercise meal Humalog by 50 percent to avoid hypoglycemia, but he continues to eat his normal amounts of food.

Diet Changes Alone

An NPH user tests his blood sugar while rock climbing on every pitch before climbing. He eats snacks as necessary to correct hypoglycemia but does not adjust his insulin doses.

Combined Insulin and Diet Changes

An NPH user finds that she can rock climb without decreasing her insulin or increasing her carbohydrate intake; however, another NPH user reduces his short-acting insulin by 1 to 2 units before starting and eats more juice and chocolate bars as needed. Another NPH user will usually reduce his regular insulin by up to 50 percent and increase his intake of simple carbohydrates when he begins climbing within an hour after a meal.

A pump user has to keep her basal rate the same while rock climbing up to eight hours or else her blood sugars rise, but she adjusts her insulin-to-carbohydrate ratio from 1:14 up to 1:30 to 1:45 (1 unit of Humalog per grams of carbohydrate). Her blood sugars tend to drop in the evening after she climbs. For indoor climbing in a gym, another pump user may cut back on his basal rate 25 percent or less, but he finds that with the intermittent, intense nature of this activity, he does not need to eat much more than usual.

An Ultralente user drastically reduces his insulin for intense all-day rock climbing. He does not take his usual basal dose of Ultralente; instead, he takes multiple injections of Regular insulin (although he usually takes Humalog) in accordance with frequent blood sugar monitoring, and he eats at least 50 percent more carbohydrate during the activity.

Intensity, Duration, and Other Effects

Effect of intensity. An NPH user finds that rock climbing is more like weight training for her, and it does not decrease her blood sugars as quickly as other activities. For climbing two to three hours after breakfast, she takes 2 to 3 units less Humalog for breakfast and 1 unit less of NPH.

Effect of duration. For rock climbing, mostly in the gym, an NPH user usually only adjusts his food intake (additional carbohydrate as needed), although he may decrease both his Regular and NPH insulin as well for daylong outdoor climbing.

MOUNTAIN BIKING

This activity is mostly a prolonged endurance sport requiring occasional bursts of anaerobic energy to climb up hills and inclines. The majority of energy comes from aerobic sources (fat and carbohydrate) with intermittent use of anaerobic systems (mainly the lactic acid system) when the intensity of exercise increases temporarily. Compensatory adjustments will depend on the terrain, which affects the intensity of biking, and the duration of the activity.

The biggest effects on all insulin regimens will be the intensity and duration of biking as well as the time of day you do the biking. More intense biking may cause blood sugars to drop less because anaerobic energy systems will be called into action, and more glucose-raising hormones will be released during the activity. The risk for hypoglycemia may actually be greater following such an intense workout than during it if circulating insulin levels are low during biking. More prolonged biking will utilize more muscle glycogen stores, resulting in a greater possibility for hypoglycemia following the activity. You will need more carbohydrate supplementation and reductions in insulin doses to prevent hypoglycemia during this period of glycogen repletion. Morning exercise will also require less regimen changes as the body is more insulin resistant at that time of day. If you exercise when circulating insulin levels are higher (within two to three hours after Humalog doses and three to four hours after regular insulin), you will usually need a greater carbohydrate intake to prevent hypoglycemia.

Athlete Examples

These examples show that mountain biking usually requires combined changes in insulin and diet together to compensate for this activity.

Diet Changes Alone

An NPH user usually bikes for 30 minutes to an hour. If his blood sugar is in the 100 to 200 mg/dl range, he finds he can usually ride without making any insulin adjustments or snacking. He eats additional carbohydrate as needed during his ride.

Combined Insulin and Diet Changes

An NPH user trains for mountain bike races. For this strenuous activity, he reduces his premeal Humalog dose by 33 to 50 percent (from 6 units to 3 or 4) and his evening NPH (the only NPH he takes) by 25 percent. He also increases his carbohydrate intake while biking and eats a bedtime snack following exercise to prevent hypoglycemia overnight.

When biking 60 minutes or more, another NPH user increases his carbohydrate and fruit intake during the activity based on the intensity of his exercise. Following the exercise, he reduces his Humalog by 1 to 2 units and decreases his bedtime Lente dose by 2 to 4 units from 18 units.

MOUNTAIN BIKING

User	Insulin	Diet
NPH/Lente	• For biking after a short-acting insulin dose, reduce the dose by 10-30% depending on the intensity of biking. • Reduce meal doses of short-acting insulin by a greater amount (30-50%) for rides lasting over an hour. • After especially prolonged or strenuous biking, reduce short-acting insulin for the following meal and evening doses of NPH or Lente by 10-30%.	• For short biking trips of less than 1 hour, make minimal increases in food intake, especially for early-morning activity or more than 3-4 hours after taking short-acting insulin (if NPH or Lente is taken at bedtime only). • Supplement with 15-30 grams or less of carbohydrate depending on the intensity of biking and the reductions in insulin. For rides lasting over an hour, eat 15-30 grams of extra carbohydrate per hour. • Eat a bedtime snack to prevent nocturnal hypoglycemia after strenuous biking.
Insulin Pump	• Reduce basal insulin rates by 15-40% during the activity and reduce preexercise meal boluses by 10-30%. • For rides lasting over an hour, reduce basal insulin rates by 25-50% during the activity and, if desired for 1-2 hours before biking. • Reduce boluses by 25-50% or take no boluses for food eaten during the activity. • Following especially prolonged or strenuous biking, reduce insulin boluses by 10-30% for the following meal. • Consider reducing basal insulin rates overnight by 10-20% following strenuous activity.	• For biking 1 hour or less, increase carbohydrate intake, especially for early-morning activity or before a meal (3-4 hours after the last insulin bolus). • Eating 15-30 grams of extra carbohydrate will usually suffice depending on the intensity of biking and reductions in insulin. • Increase carbohydrate intake by 15-30 grams per hour for longer rides. • Eat a bedtime snack to prevent overnight hypoglycemia after prolonged biking.
Ultralente	• Reduce short-acting insulin by 10-30% for meals before biking. • Reduce morning Ultralente doses by 10-20% in anticipation of prolonged biking of 2 hours or more, and reduce preactivity meal insulin by 25-50%. • Following prolonged or strenuous biking, reduce doses of short-acting insulin by 10-30% for the next meal. • Consider a reduction in the evening Ultralente doses of 10-20% if biking was prolonged or very strenuous.	• For short biking trips of less than 1 hour, make minimal increases in food intake, especially for early-morning activity or when circulating insulin levels are low. • An intake of 15-30 grams of extra carbohydrate will usually suffice depending on the intensity of biking. • For rides lasting more than an hour, increase carbohydrate intake by 15-30 grams per hour or more. • Eat a bedtime snack to prevent overnight hypoglycemia if the activity was strenuous or prolonged.

A pump user tries to reduce the amount of Regular insulin circulating in his body during mountain biking by reducing his pump basal rate from 0.7 units per hour to 0.4 for two to three hours before biking. If he eats before starting, he tries to eat at least two hours before and takes a Humalog bolus only (no Regular insulin) of no more than 1.5 units. If he eats and then exercises right away, he does not take a meal bolus but will take a reduced bolus after the exercise. For early-morning exercise, he makes less of a reduction in his basal rate (to 0.5) or no reduction.

Another pump user decreases the basal rate on her pump from 0.5 units per hour to 0.3 units normally, or to 0.2 units for riding uphill, for mountain biking from 90 minutes to five hours. She is able to eat more carbohydrate for the same Humalog bolus (1 unit for 30 to 45 grams of carbohydrate instead of the usual 14 grams per unit). If she exercises more than four hours, she reduces her basal rate at night by 0.1 units per hour and eats a larger snack before going to bed.

An Ultralente user decreases her morning Ultralente dose by 1 unit for every hour of biking and her Humalog by 2 units before exercise and supplements with 15 grams of carbohydrate every 20 to 30 minutes based on the intensity of her riding.

Intensity, Duration, and Other Effects

Effect of duration and intensity. An NPH user bikes for 30 to 60 minutes without making any insulin adjustments or snacking if his starting blood sugar is in the 100 to 200 mg/dl range. A pump user finds that she needs less food for mountain biking than for regular road biking due to the more intense nature of mountain biking.

Effect of time of day. A bedtime-only NPH user either mountain bikes 15 to 20 miles (light days) or 20 to 30 miles (heavy days) early in the morning before taking any insulin. If his blood sugar is between 70 and 130 mg/dl, he does not make any dietary adjustments. For blood sugar of 140 or higher, he takes a small amount of Humalog and waits for it to take effect before biking.

HORSEBACK RIDING

This activity is usually low-intensity and aerobic. It uses a lot of postural muscles to keep on top of the horse while it is moving. The faster the horse is going, the more energy required to hold on and stay on. Recreational riding will generally not affect blood sugar levels, and minimal regimen changes will be necessary. A longer duration (all-day trail rides) or a higher intensity of riding may have a bigger effect on blood sugars, and some slight reductions in insulin doses or increases in carbohydrate intake may be necessary to prevent hypoglycemia.

Athlete Examples

Due to the low intensity of this activity, most people make adjustments with diet alone or with very small changes in their insulin doses.

Diet Changes Alone

Normally an NPH user makes no insulin adjustments for one to two hours of hard riding, but she may decrease her insulin slightly for an all-day horse competition. She supplements with snacks as needed to raise her blood sugar to 170 mg/dl to prevent hypoglycemia during 60 minutes of horseback riding. For occasional recreational riding, a pump user makes no adjustments to her basal rate or boluses. She checks her blood sugar occasionally during her ride and may snack if needed.

Combined Insulin and Diet Changes

For 90-minute rides, an NPH user does not make any adjustments to her insulin or food intake. Another NPH user may reduce his regular insulin by 1 unit for this activity or eat an extra snack of up to 200 calories if needed.

SKYDIVING

This activity requires very little energy, mainly muscular contractions on impact with the ground. It may, however, cause an increase in anxiety and release of epinephrine (adrenaline), which can raise blood sugar levels. Skydivers will need to monitor their blood sugars before and after diving. If blood sugar levels increase, an additional dose of short-acting insulin may be necessary to compensate for the rise (about 1 unit for each 50 mg/dl increase). Neither decreases in insulin nor increases in food intake for this activity are generally advised.

CANOEING AND KAYAKING

Canoeing and kayaking are prolonged and aerobic in nature, especially at lower intensities. The body mainly uses fat and carbohydrate, and carbohydrate use increases with exercise intensity. Whitewater activities can be more intense and cause a greater use of anaerobic energy sources such as the lactic acid system. The more prolonged the activity (especially if intense), the more regimen adjustments you will need to maintain blood sugar levels. You can modify insulin doses, food intake, or both depending on the exercise intensity and duration.

The intensity and duration of canoeing and kayaking have the biggest effects on blood sugars. For low-level paddling, you will need minimal changes. For longer or more intense paddling, you may need more food and insulin changes to prevent hypoglycemia. For multiple-day trips, you may need reductions in longer-acting or basal rates of insulin (10 to 20 percent) because more glycogen depletion will occur in the upper-body muscles.

Athlete Examples

These examples show changes in diet, insulin, and both, depending on the intensity, duration, and timing of the canoeing or kayaking.

Insulin Changes Alone

For low-intensity daylong canoe trips, an NPH user slightly decreases her Humalog doses by 1 unit during the day. She takes NPH only at bedtime, and she does not adjust this dose. For 60 minutes of canoeing, a pump user usually reduces her basal rate by 0.2 units per hour (from 0.7 to 0.5). If she does the activity immediately after breakfast, she may also lower her prebreakfast bolus slightly. During four hours of canoeing, another pump user disconnects her pump, but her blood sugar usually increases to 200 mg/dl. She then boluses 1 to 2 units of Humalog when she reconnects her pump.

CANOEING AND KAYAKING

User	Insulin*	Diet
NPH/Lente	• Reduce preactivity short-acting insulin doses by 10-20% for canoeing lasting over an hour, and reduce morning NPH by the same amount for all-day or afternoon activity. • For more intense and prolonged activities like sea kayaking or white-water canoeing, reduce insulin by 20-40% and moderately increase carbohydrate intake. • No changes in bedtime doses of NPH or Lente are usually necessary, except after especially prolonged activity or multiple-day trips.	• Eat 0-10 grams of carbohydrate per hour for low-level canoeing, • For more intense paddling, eat 10-20 grams of carbohydrates per hour depending on the actual insulin reductions.
Insulin Pump	• Reduce basal insulin rates by 25-50% during the activity depending on the intensity. • Reduce preactivity meal boluses by 10-20% for less intense activities, and reduce them by 20-40% for more intense or prolonged paddling. • Complete removal of the pump may work for short-duration paddling, but removing the pump for more than 2 hours may result in hyperglycemia. • Temporarily reduce basal insulin rates overnight by 10-20% following prolonged activity or multiple-day trips.	• Increase carbohydrate intake depending on the reduction in basal rates and meal boluses. • For low-level canoeing, make minimal increases of 0-10 grams of carbohydrate per hour along with reductions in insulin. • For more intense paddling, eat about 10-20 grams of carbohydrate per hour.
Ultralente	• Reduce preactivity short-acting insulin dose by 10-20% for shorter, less intense activity. • Reduce short-acting insulin dose by 20-40% for more prolonged or intense activity. • Do not alter Ultralente doses except possibly for especially prolonged or multiple-day canoeing.	• Depending on the reductions in short-acting insulin and the intensity and duration of paddling, make small to moderate increases in carbohydrate intake. • Increase carbohydrates by 0-10 grams per hour for low-level canoeing. • Increase by 10-20 grams for more intense paddling.

* The length and intensity of the activity will determine the necessary changes. For shorter, less intense activities, make very small (if any) modifications in insulin.

Diet Changes Alone

For moderate canoeing with his children, an NPH user just eats additional carbohydrate as needed during the activity. For canoeing one to two hours at a time, an Ultralente user supplements with additional carbohydrate and water as needed. For white-water canoeing and kayaking, another NPH user simply increases her intake of snacks, dried fruit, and cheese and crackers. For sea kayaking, another NPH user makes sure that his blood sugar is not dropping and that it is somewhat elevated (150 to 200 mg/dl) when he starts this activity. To do so, he supplements with additional carbohydrates before and during the activity as needed.

Combined Insulin and Diet Changes

Before canoeing, an NPH user either reduces his regular insulin by 1 to 2 units or he eats 200 to 300 more calories. For canoeing in the early morning, another NPH user will reduce or eliminate her prebreakfast Humalog (usually 2 units) but take her usual morning dose of NPH. She supplements with additional food as needed for prolonged paddling. Another NPH user undertakes one- to two-day white-water canoeing trips in a two-person canoe. She only cuts her Humalog dose during the day minimally (by 10 to 15 percent per meal) and may eat a few extra carbohydrates.

A pump user finds that she needs to decrease her basal rate by 50 percent about 30 minutes before canoeing and keep it reduced for the duration of the exercise (down from 1.1 units per hour). She drinks four ounces of juice before canoeing if her blood sugar is 100 mg/dl or lower. Another pump user usually leaves his basal rate the same for canoeing and kayaking and balances his blood sugars with extra carbohydrate. If he eats a meal before canoeing, he takes only a small Humalog dose to cover the meal and tries to begin exercising at least two hours after eating when the effects of the Humalog are minimized.

An Ultralente user decreases his Humalog dose by 50 percent for this activity. He monitors his blood sugar and snacks frequently while canoeing.

Intensity, Duration, and Other Effects

Effect of intensity. An Ultralente user canoes and white-water rafts down a river for two to six hours at a time. When she begins her activity after breakfast, she usually reduces her prebreakfast Humalog dose by 20 percent as well as her prelunch dose. She tries to eat a large meal for breakfast because upper-body exercise reduces her blood sugars quite quickly. She eats granola bars that she carries in resealable plastic bags. For blood sugars below 120 mg/dl, she will drink 12 ounces of soda or six ounces of juice.

Effect of time of day. An NPH user found that during a channel crossing under adverse conditions in the morning when insulin resistance is highest, his blood sugars remained normal with no insulin or breakfast before the activity.

Effect of multiple days of activity. For canoeing trips lasting three days, an NPH user reduces her insulin from 23/6 (NPH/regular) to 18 to 20 units of NPH and 4 units of Regular in the morning. In the evening she reduces her NPH by 1 to 2 units and her regular by 1 (from 3 to 2). She also eats more food while paddling, especially for breakfast, lunch, and snacks.

WINDSURFING

This activity usually involves prolonged muscular contractions that involve holding onto the sail and stabilizing your body on the board. Windsurfing is a lot like isometric resistance training, which uses static muscle contractions. You will mainly use anaerobic energy sources, but aerobic energy derived from carbohydrate and fat will also fuel these sustained contractions of postural muscles. The intensity and duration of this activity will depend on wind conditions and your skill level. You can maintain blood sugars through changes in insulin doses, food intake, or both, depending mainly on how long you do the activity and the prevailing wind conditions, both of which affect intensity of the exercise.

The biggest effect on blood sugar levels for windsurfing comes from the prevailing wind conditions. Stronger winds will increase the exercise intensity and carbohydrate use during the activity (both from blood glucose and muscle glycogen sources). You may need adjustments in both insulin and food intake under these conditions if you windsurf for more than 30 minutes at a time. Lighter winds will cause greater fat utilization during the activity and a reduced use of blood glucose and muscle glycogen stores.

Athlete Examples

These examples show that the regimen changes largely depend on the wind conditions and the duration of the activity.

Insulin Changes Alone

A pump user usually windsurfs on a lake for 30 to 45 minutes. He checks his blood sugar before going out. If blood sugars are on

WINDSURFING

User	Insulin	Diet
NPH/Lente	• For light winds or short-duration windsurfing, reduce short-acting insulin at the preceding meal by 10-25%. • For stronger winds or longer durations, reduce short-acting insulin doses by 15-40%. • For windsurfing done in the afternoon, reduce morning NPH doses (if taken) by 10-25%.	• Eat 10-15 grams of extra carbohydrate per hour for this activity if insulin is not reduced. • Supplement with up to 30 grams of carbohydrate per hour or more for windsurfing if insulin is peaking or for stronger winds or longer durations.
Insulin Pump	• For shorter-duration surfing or lighter winds, reduce basal rates by 25-50% or remove the insulin pump altogether. • Take an additional bolus when reconnecting the pump if blood sugars have risen. • Reduce boluses by 10-25% for meals before the activity. • For longer durations or higher winds, remove the pump during the activity and reduce preactivity boluses by 15-40%.	• With basal insulin reductions, make minimal carbohydrate increases during most windsurfing. • Supplement with up to 15-30 grams of carbohydrate per hour to prevent hypoglycemia during longer durations or higher winds.
Ultralente	• For shorter durations or lighter winds, reduce insulin by 10-25%. • For longer durations or higher winds, reduce insulin by 15-40%.	• If windsurfing when circulating insulin levels are low, you will need minimal carbohydrate supplementation. • Increase carbohydrate intake by up to 15-30 grams per hour depending on the duration of the activity and prevailing wind conditions.

the low side or they are falling, he will not go out on the lake until they have stabilized. If the wind is light to moderate, he wears his pump in a sport case and maintains his basal rate of insulin. If the winds are high, he disconnects the pump and takes a bolus when he reconnects to cover for the missed insulin.

Diet Changes Alone

For windsurfing, an NPH user makes sure that his blood sugar is not dropping and that it is somewhat elevated (150 to 200 mg/dl) when he starts this activity for two to four hours. He supplements with additional carbohydrate before and during the activity as needed.

Combined Insulin and Diet Changes

An NPH user finds that it is difficult to predict the wind conditions before going out on the water. Therefore, she usually does not reduce her Humalog insulin, but instead she will eat extra carbohydrate while sailing depending on the wind conditions. If she can reduce her insulin in advance, she cuts her Humalog at the preceding meal by 25 to 30 percent for a difficult sail with strong wind conditions and tries to begin with a blood sugar level of 140 mg/dl or higher.

SURFING AND BOOGIEBOARDING

Surfing and boogieboarding are both anaerobic and aerobic in nature. Both require using muscles, usually postural muscles, which are more aerobic in nature, to maintain balance while riding a wave. The anaerobic component is utilized by the quick recruitment of additional muscles to maintain balance and adjust to changes in the waves, especially while surfing. The duration of each ride can be rather short, making the activity more intermittent than continuous. When you paddle out to meet a wave, you tend to rely more on anaerobic energy sources because of the shortness of the activity. You can regulate the effects of these activities on blood sugar with changes in diet, insulin, or both, depending on your insulin regimen, the duration of the activity, and size and roughness of the waves.

SURFING AND BOOGIEBOARDING*

User	Insulin	Diet
NPH/Lente	• For surfing closely following a meal, reduce short-acting insulin doses by 20-50% depending on planned surfing duration and intensity. • Reduce morning NPH doses (if taken) by 10-30% for afternoon or prolonged exercise. • If insulin doses are reduced only a small amount under these conditions, eat additional carbohydrate. • At other times when circulating insulin is lower, make minimal changes in insulin unless the activity is prolonged or waves are rough.	• For surfing when insulin doses are peaking, eat an additional 15-30 grams of carbohydrate per hour (following a meal or in the afternoon if morning NPH is taken). • When circulating insulin levels are lower, Increase carbohydrate intake minimally unless the activity is prolonged or waves are rough.
Insulin Pump	• Remove insulin pump during this activity or reduce the basal rate of insulin by 25-50%. • Take a supplemental bolus when reconnecting the pump if disconnected for an hour or more and blood sugars begin to rise. • For surfing closely following a meal, reduce insulin boluses by 20-50% depending on the planned duration and intensity of the activity.	• Eat an extra 15-30 grams of carbohydrate per hour depending on the reductions in insulin and the ocean wave conditions.
Ultralente	• For surfing closely following a meal, reduce short-acting insulin doses by 20-50% depending on wave size. • If the activity is done more than 3-4 hours following the last dose of short-acting insulin, then make no insulin changes.	• Eat an additional 15-30 grams of carbohydrate per hour for surfing within 3-4 hours of the last injection of short-acting insulin or when ocean conditions are rougher. • When circulating insulin levels are lower, minimal carbohydrate supplementation may be necessary unless this surfing is prolonged or intense.

* Surfing on larger, more vigorous waves will have greater glucose-reducing effects and require bigger insulin reductions and/or food increases.

The intensity of surfing and boogieboarding has the greatest potential effect on blood sugars, which will be largely determined by the ocean conditions. Riding waves for a longer period at a higher intensity will generally reduce blood sugars more than doing these activities under calmer conditions. You will need greater regimen changes for these rougher conditions.

Athlete Examples

These examples show that you can manage this activity with any type of regimen change (diet, insulin, or both).

Insulin Changes Alone

A Lente user reduces his Lente and Humalog doses by 30 percent for surfing. He supplements with carbohydrate only if he needs to. An NPH user usually takes only 50 percent of his usual Humalog for the meal before this exercise and drinks juice while exercising if needed.

Diet Changes Alone

For this activity, an Ultralente user usually does not adjust his insulin doses. He carries a PowerBar in his wetsuit to eat if needed.

Combined Insulin and Diet Changes

A pump user may reduce his basal rate by 20 to 25 percent and supplement with additional carbohydrate as needed. He also makes sure that his infusion site is far on the side of his abdomen, or he disconnects the pump for up to an hour while doing the activity and takes an extra bolus when he reconnects based on his blood sugar.

SCUBA DIVING

Scuba diving is mainly a low-intensity aerobic activity involving slow kicking and some arm movements. The main concern is the effect of the high environmental pressure experienced underwater: it can increase the rate of absorption of insulin from subcutaneous injection sites and cause an underwater hypoglycemic reaction, which may go unrecognized or be difficult to treat.

Historically, people with type 1 diabetes and other insulin users have not been allowed to obtain National Association of Underwater Instructors (NAUI) certifications to allow them to legally scuba dive (although Professional Association of Diving Instructors, or PADI, may be obtainable) due to NAUI's fear of untreatable hypoglycemic episodes occurring during diving. Also, the increase in intraocular (eye) pressures may also worsen diabetic eye disease or cause retinal hemorrhaging. However, many people have dived safely anyway. In response to the actions of these people, the Divers' Alert Network (DAN) has conducted several studies on the safety of diving for people with diabetes. As a result, a move to allow more widely available diving accreditation for people with type 1 diabetes is under way, and guidelines for safe diving are being established.

Steve Prosterman, an athlete with type 1 diabetes, runs an outdoor activity camp that includes scuba-diving camp (Camp DAVI) in the U.S. Virgin Islands for diabetic people (see profile in chapter 4). He stresses the importance of glucose monitoring to determine whether glucose levels are stable, rising, or falling before diving. He has divers test 60 minutes, 30 minutes, and immediately before diving. If their blood sugar levels are stable, then he has them aim for a slightly higher than normal level (150 to 180 mg/dl) before diving. If their blood sugars are rising, then he sets a minimum level of 140 to 150 mg/dl as desirable. According to his recommendations, under no circumstances should a person dive if his or her blood sugar is dropping. A diver should ingest carbohydrates until blood sugar is stable or rising. His guidelines also include carrying some form of waterproof glucose that can be ingested on the surface, such as glucose gels, honey, or cake frosting; being able to recognize and treat hypoglycemia; having no advanced secondary diabetic complications (especially active eye disease); and diving with a buddy educated in diabetes. If hypoglycemia occurs, the person gives an "L" signal to his buddy with his thumb and forefinger, and both divers surface. A dive depth limit of 90 feet (27 meters) is recommended to help rule out confusion between nitrogen narcosis and low blood sugar symptoms. Decompression diving, which is diving to great depth or for a more extended period of time requiring a very slow ascent to the surface, is never done in case hypoglycemia would occur and require surfacing. He also recommends being conservative with the dive tables as some evidence suggests that diabetic people may be more prone to dehydration (implicated in decompression sickness, "the bends") while diving.

Increased pressure in an underwater environment and the water temperature are the biggest potential effects of scuba diving on blood sugar levels. Increased pressure can speed the absorption of insulin that you inject subcutaneously. As a result, large increases in the levels of circulating insulin can occur, especially if you have injected short-acting insulins within three to four hours of a dive. Increased absorption rates of longer-acting insulins (NPH, Lente, and Ultralente) can also occur. Injecting lower doses of or no insulin before dives can help minimize these effects. The water temperature can also affect energy expenditure. Colder water will increase the metabolic rate while diving, even if you wear a wetsuit, and may require greater changes in insulin or diet before diving than warmer ocean conditions.

Athlete Examples

The following examples show that most people attempt to reduce their circulating levels of insulin during a dive by taking less short-acting insulin before the activity. There is also an example of the dramatic effects of the environmental conditions.

Insulin Changes Alone

A Lente user reduces both of his insulins, Lente and Humalog, by 30 percent as a precaution before scuba diving. An Ultralente user decreases his morning Ultralente dose by 1 to 2 units, takes little or no Humalog before diving, and has a sport drink available to treat hypoglycemia.

Diet Changes Alone

An NPH user tests her blood sugar 90 minutes before diving to monitor whether her blood sugar is rising or falling. To ensure that it is rising, she usually snacks before the dive then tests her blood sugar levels again immediately before diving to ensure that her sugars stay high enough for the duration of the dive.

Combined Insulin and Diet Changes

An evening NPH user takes no Regular insulin before morning dives unless her blood sugar is higher than 300 mg/dl, and she drinks a regular soda between dives. Another NPH user takes 50 percent less Regular in the morning (from 9 units to 4.5 units) and 20 percent less NPH on a dive day (down from her usual morning dose of 11). She eats according to her blood sugar tests before and after a dive.

For morning dives, an Ultralente user eats a big breakfast and reduces her premeal Humalog by 20 percent. She checks her blood sugar before she goes out on the dive boat and 10 to 15 minutes before going down. If she does two dives, she checks again, and if her sugar is below 150 mg/dl, she eats half of a peanut butter and jelly sandwich before her second dive. Another Ultralente user reduces his premeal Humalog by 50 percent before dives and then eats a candy bar before each dive to prevent hypoglycemia.

A pump user disconnects his pump at the start of a dive. He tries to start with his blood sugar in the 150 to 180 mg/dl range. He checks his blood sugar and eats additional carbohydrate as needed after every 30 to 45 minutes of diving. He never dives for longer than 45 minutes due to the large drops in blood sugar levels that he experiences with longer dives.

Intensity, Duration, and Other Effects

Effect of environment. An NPH user varies her regimen depending on where she dives. When diving in the cold Atlantic Ocean, she wears a wetsuit. Under these conditions, she will not enter the water unless her blood glucose is more than 150 mg/dl. She eats a granola bar before the dive and tries to keep her blood sugar at 180 or above. She also reduces her breakfast Humalog by 50 percent and her lunch dose by 80 percent. After her second dive in the afternoon, she needs to take some additional Humalog or her blood sugars will begin to rise. In contrast, for diving in warm waters in the Caribbean, she does not need a wetsuit, and her dives are shallower. She will often enter the water with her blood sugar between 80 and 100 mg/dl as long as she is sure that it is rising. She reduces her insulin doses minimally under these conditions.

SNORKELING

Snorkeling is a low-intensity aerobic exercise. It is slower and less intense than regular swimming because you do not use your upper

SNORKELING

User	Insulin	Diet
NPH/Lente	• For less than 1 hour of snorkeling, modify insulin doses minimally (0-10%). • Reduce short-acting insulin doses by 0-20% for snorkeling lasting over an hour; reduce morning NPH (if taken) by the same amount for all-day or afternoon activity. • For more prolonged activity, reduce short-acting insulin by 10-30%. • Bedtime doses of NPH or Lente should remain the same.	• Increase carbohydrate by up to 15 grams per hour depending on the reductions in insulin for snorkeling more than an hour. • For more prolonged snorkeling, eat 10-30 extra grams of carbohydrate per hour if insulin is not sufficiently reduced.
Insulin Pump	• Reduce basal insulin rates by 0-100% during the activity, depending on the intensity. • If the insulin pump is not water-proof, remove it while snorkeling. • Reduce preactivity meal boluses by 0-20% for shorter durations and by 10-30% for longer durations. Less of a reduction is necessary if pump is removed during snorkeling. • Complete removal of the pump may work for short durations but may result in hyperglycemia after a couple of hours. • Take a supplemental bolus when reconnecting the pump if discon-nected for an hour or more and blood sugars begin to rise.	• Increase carbohydrate intake depending on the reduction in basal rates and meal boluses. • Increase carbohydrate intake by 0-10 grams per hour for shorter durations, and by 10-20 grams per hour for prolonged snorkeling.
Ultralente	• Reduce short-acting insulin doses by 0-20% for shorter-duration snorkeling. • Reduce short-acting insulin doses by a greater amount (10-30%) for more prolonged snorkeling. • No change in Ultralente doses is generally necessary.	• Make small to moderate increases in carbohydrate intake depending on the intensity and duration of the activity. • Eat 0-15 grams per hour for shorter durations and 10-30 grams per hour of extra carbohydrate for longer durations.

body as much, but kicking with swim fins provides greater resistance for your legs. The intensity can vary somewhat with your kicking speed and interspersed periods of floating and minimal kicking. Due to its low intensity, you will need minimal regimen changes to maintain blood sugars effectively.

The duration of snorkeling has the biggest effect on blood sugar control. For short durations you will need minimal changes. You may need increased food intake and insulin reductions for longer durations to prevent hypoglycemia. The intensity of snorkeling can also vary with kicking speed. For higher intensities, expect a larger drop in blood sugars and make appropriate regimen adjustments.

Athlete Examples

These real-life examples show that you can make minor adjustments in diet or insulin alone to compensate for the effects of snorkeling.

Insulin Changes Alone

A pump user finds that snorkeling requires no major adjustments in her insulin dose or carbohydrate intake. If she does this activity for less than an hour, she removes her pump. If she snorkels for a longer period of time, she usually keeps her pump on but decreases her basal rate by 10 to 20 percent. Another pump user varies her regimen according to her snorkeling intensity. If the intensity is low, she needs almost no insulin or food intake adjustments. If she swims hard while snorkeling, she decreases both her preexercise meal bolus and her basal rate by 50 percent during the activity. An Ultralente user may decrease his Humalog dose if the snorkeling is prolonged.

Diet Changes Alone

For mild-intensity snorkeling, an NPH user does not make any changes in her insulin. She checks her blood sugar often and snacks often during the activity.

WATERSKIING, JETSKIING, AND SNOWMOBILING

All of these activities are anaerobic in nature because they involve prolonged muscular contractions (holding onto the rope and stabilizing your body on the skis during waterskiing, for example). The intensity and duration of these activities can affect blood sugar response, especially if the activity becomes more aerobic as the duration increases. You can alter food intake and insulin, but you will usually need minimal changes due to the brief, intense nature of these activities. If you do these activities after a meal, you may reduce doses of short-acting insulin by 10 to 20 percent or not at all, but you will not need to alter carbohydrate intake if you reduce insulin. If you are a pump user, you may remove your pump during this activity and take a supplemental bolus later if you keep your pump disconnected for an hour or more.

The intensity of waterskiing, jetskiing, and snowmobiling has the greatest potential effect on blood sugars. Blood sugars are usually more effectively maintained during short, high-intensity activities because they result in a greater release of hormones that increase blood sugar levels. Hypoglycemia is less likely to result from anaerobic activities than more prolonged aerobic activities, so you will need fewer regimen adjustments.

Athlete Examples

An NPH user only makes adjustments for waterskiing based on her starting blood sugar. If her blood sugar is in the 140 to 160 mg/dl range before beginning, she makes no adjustments; if it is below that range, she may have a small snack, and if higher, she may take a small amount of Humalog insulin. An insulin pump user takes his pump off during waterskiing but makes no other adjustments to his diet or insulin unless he becomes hypoglycemic.

SAILING

Sailing is mainly anaerobic, requiring short bursts of powerful movements such as pulling a rope, with little movement between pulls except for the work of postural muscles to maintain balance while standing on the deck. The intensity may vary with the size of the boat, the number of crew members, and the strength of the wind. Regimen changes depend on the conditions that affect the intensity of sailing.

For normal recreational sailing, you will usually need no changes in insulin or food intake. For intensive sailing involving more physical labor, you can reduce short-acting insulin doses by 10 to 25 percent, either alone or with an increase in carbohydrates of 10 to 15 grams per hour.

The intensity of sailing has the biggest effect on blood sugar response. Strong wind conditions may not affect larger boats, and larger boats may also carry more crew members. With fewer crew members, each sailor has to do more work. Stronger winds will also require more effort and more directional changes to control the boat.

Athlete Examples

These real-life examples show that the level of competition has a big effect on regimen changes, but most sailing will require few changes.

Insulin Changes Alone

For weekend boating, an Ultralente user decreases his doses by 1 to 2 units and takes little or no Humalog before and during the activity. He also has sport drinks available to treat hypoglycemia.

Diet Changes Alone

An NPH user finds that crewing on a racing boat once a week does not require much physical labor. Therefore, she does not change her insulin or her carbohydrate intake. She does bring her insulin, blood glucose meter, and extra food with her. A pump user tests his blood sugar before sailing, hourly while sailing, and afterward and takes glucose tablets for fine-tuning his blood sugars. An Ultralente user, however, finds sailing to be a surprising amount of exercise. He usually takes his normal insulin doses of Humalog and Ultralente but increases his usual carbohydrate intake by 50 percent during the activity.

Combined Insulin and Diet Changes

An NPH user considers sailing a light activity. He may reduce his regular insulin by up to 1 unit or eat up to 200 calories extra for the activity. An insulin pump user participates in offshore sailing and racing. For a full day of this activity, he consumes extra apple juice, fruits, granola, food bars, raisins, and peanut butter crackers. Usually he maintains the basal rate on his pump but reduces his boluses while sailing and constantly snacks to maintain his blood sugar around 140 mg/dl. He finds he uses extra energy just trying to maintain his balance in heavy seas. An Ultralente user sails recreationally on a 14-foot sailboat. For sailing two hours in a regatta, she reduces her lunch Humalog dose by 20 percent. She eats a Snickers bar near the end of the two-hour regatta on windy days only.

Intensity, Duration, and Other Effects

Effect of competition. For competitive sailboat racing with a crew of four to six people, an NPH user tries to keep his blood sugars perfect. He decreases his Humalog dose by 10 to 40 percent for this activity. He monitors his blood sugars and snacks as needed between sail changes. When he skippers the boat, he finds this activity to be less physically demanding. In close races, stress can increase his blood sugar levels dramatically.

BEACH VOLLEYBALL

This activity involves only short, powerful moves such as serving or hitting the ball and is anaerobic in nature. It utilizes more energy than volleyball on a regular court, though, because much more energy is utilized to walk or run on sand. Recreational play can involve minimal activity as players are not involved actively in every play, and moving to and hitting the ball require only short bursts of activity. Fewer players or more competitive or longer games may affect blood sugar levels more. For specific recommendations for a comparable sport, refer to the section on volleyball in chapter 8.

DOWNHILL SKIING AND SNOWBOARDING

These activities use a mix of anaerobic and aerobic fuels, depending on skiing or snowboarding techniques. A skilled skier on more difficult slopes may use more energy by skiing intensely. Snow conditions (powdery versus icy) and the temperature and wind chill on the slopes also affect fuel use. The skiing and environmental conditions, as well as skill level of the skier, will dictate regimen changes on a given day.

The regimen changes required for downhill skiing and snowboarding will depend on the skier's skill level, duration of skiing, and environmental conditions. People who are constantly shifting and moving while skiing engage in a more aerobic activity, which will use more fuels including muscle glycogen and blood glucose. Skiing straight downhill and letting gravity do most of the work requires minimal energy expenditure and will, accordingly, have a minimal effect on blood sugars. Spending time in chairlift lines, on the chairlift, or in the lodge warming up will also reduce overall energy expenditure. Intense skiing at a higher skill level or for a

DOWNHILL SKIING AND SNOWBOARDING

User	Insulin*	Diet
NPH/Lente	• For all-day or more intense skiing, reduce premeal doses of short-acting insulin by 20-30%. • Reduce morning doses of NPH (if taken) by 20-30% for afternoon activity.	• Supplement with 15 grams of carbohydrate or less per hour for more intense skiing.
Insulin Pump	• Reduce premeal boluses by 10-30% for all-day or more intense skiing or snowboarding. • Reduce basal insulin rates by 25-50% as well during the activity.	• If necessary, consume 10-15 grams of additional carbohydrate per hour.
Ultralente	• For all-day or more intense activities, reduce doses of short-acting insulin by 10-30% for meals.	• If necessary, consume up to 10-15 grams of extra carbohydrate per hour during the activity.

* Make minimal changes in insulin doses for shorter-duration skiing (less than 1-2 hours). Very cold or windy conditions may have a greater blood-glucose lowering effect.

prolonged time will increase energy expenditure as well. More powdery snow can make skiing more difficult and require more energy compared to slopes covered with a sheet of ice. Colder weather or a more severe wind chill factor can also increase the amount of energy used by the body just to stay warm.

Athlete Examples

The reported regimen changes vary widely with the intensity and duration of skiing or snowboarding as well as the environmental conditions. Some people make insulin changes, others change their food intake, some do neither, and some do both.

Insulin Changes Alone

For skiing, an NPH user decreases her Humalog during the day by 15 to 20 percent, but she makes no modifications in her diet. For all-day aggressive skiing, another NPH user may reduce her morning NPH dose by 20 percent and supplement with snacks as needed during the day. For high-intensity skiing, a Lente user reduces both his Humalog and Lente doses by 50 percent.

A pump user decreases the basal rate on her pump by 25 percent while skiing. She finds it difficult to predict her blood sugar response because skiing is such an intermittent activity. An Ultralente user reduces his Humalog doses for his normal meals by 50 percent while downhill skiing.

Diet Changes Alone

For six hours of downhill skiing, an NPH user does not make any adjustments to his insulin (regular and Humalog combined during the day and NPH at bedtime only). He eats extra carbohydrate before and during the exercise. Another NPH user skis from when the lifts open until they close with one hour off for lunch. For this activity, she makes no major changes in her insulin dose. She may decrease her morning Regular insulin by 1 unit, but she snacks on M&M's. She has a handful or two every other ski run in the morning and much fewer in the afternoon, only one to two handfuls total.

A pump user keeps her basal rate normal for downhill skiing, or else her sugars begin to rise. She is able to eat two to three times more carbohydrates for the same Humalog bolus while actively skiing.

Combined Insulin and Diet Changes

An NPH user used to reduce his Regular dose for skiing at the expert level but that caused hyperglycemia. Now he does not make any adjustments to his insulin dose. For downhill skiing, another NPH user checks his blood sugar and increases his food intake by about 25 percent and reduces his morning NPH by about 30 to 40 percent (normally 14 units). For snowboarding or downhill skiing, a bedtime-only Lente user reduces his Humalog intake during the activity and supplements with more food or candy as required to maintain his blood sugar levels.

For downhill skiing, a pump user finds that she needs to make no adjustments to her insulin or diet during this activity, while another pump user decreases his insulin by 10 percent and increases his carbohydrate intake by 10 percent for downhill skiing. Another pump user reduces her basal rate by 50 to 60 percent for downhill skiing lasting five to six hours. She checks her blood sugar every two to three hours and maintains her blood sugars above 130 mg/dl with snacks if necessary. For snowboarding, a pump user decreases his basal rate by 25 percent and checks his blood sugar frequently. He snacks on trail mix or raisins to maintain his blood sugar.

For downhill skiing, an Ultralente user makes no adjustments in her insulin or diet. For moderate-intensity downhill skiing, another Ultralente user reduces his Humalog doses by 5 to 10 percent at each meal during the activity and also supplements with carbohydrates depending on his blood sugar levels.

Intensity, Duration, and Other Effects

Effect of intensity. A bedtime-only NPH user trains seriously for downhill ski racing. For training or racing, he reduces his premeal Humalog by 33 to 50 percent (from 6 units to 3 or 4) and also reduces his bedtime NPH by 25 percent. He always carries M&M's with him and eats five to six of them every chairlift ride or two. For moderate skiing, a pump user makes little or no adjustments to his insulin or diet, but for aggressive skiing, he disconnects his pump during the activity. For downhill ski racing, an Ultralente user finds that she actually must increase her Humalog insulin following this activity because her blood sugars increase.

Effect of environmental conditions. An NPH user usually eats more while skiing as she does sense her low blood sugars as well in the cold. However, she does not adjust her insulin for this activity. Another NPH user finds that skiing causes greater fluctuations in her blood sugar levels because of the altitude. She reduces her prebreakfast regular but takes the same amount of NPH in the morning before skiing. A pump user finds that she usually does not need to make any diet or insulin adjustments for downhill skiing, but if she skis in deep, heavy snow that makes her work harder, she eats extra carbohydrates.

Effect of time of day. A bedtime-only NPH user varies her regimen depending on the time of day she skis. For morning skiing, she decreases her morning short-acting insulin by 1 unit and increases her carbohydrate intake during the activity. In the afternoon, she takes more insulin and eats less carbohydrate. An Ultralente user either skis for three to four hours in the morning or for two hours before dinner on the intermediate or expert slopes. For skiing in the morning, she reduces her morning Humalog dose by 20 percent and eats a Snickers bar about midmorning. For late-afternoon skiing, she eats two ounces of cheese before she skis for two hours if her blood sugar is 120 mg/dl or lower and eats dinner right after.

SNOWSHOEING

This activity is mainly aerobic. Snowshoeing is usually slower than regular walking, but it can be more intense than walking or hiking due to the resistance of pulling the snowshoe out of the snow with each step, especially if the snow is powdery. The terrain is similar to that for hiking, backpacking, or cross-country skiing. Changes in insulin and diet will depend on the duration of this activity as well as the environmental conditions. For specific regimen changes, refer to the recommendations in the section on hiking earlier in this chapter.

Regimen changes for this activity will depend largely on the duration of snowshoeing and the environmental conditions. The intensity of snowshoeing can be greater than hiking, especially in powdery snow that is more difficult to walk in. Environmental conditions, mainly high altitude and low temperatures, affect blood sugar as well. These conditions decrease insulin needs as they increase the body's energy expenditure and blood glucose utilization, resulting in a higher risk of hypoglycemia.

Athlete Examples

For most people engaging in moderate snowshoeing, a combination of diet and insulin changes appears to work best to maintain blood sugars.

Insulin Changes Alone

A pump user only makes insulin adjustments when she does this activity after a meal. She reduces her premeal bolus before engaging in the activity.

Diet Changes Alone

A pump user finds that for every 20 to 30 minutes of snowshoeing, she needs to eat an additional 30 grams of carbohydrate. Sometimes she drinks juice that is 50 percent diluted or takes glucose tablets. Another pump user does not adjust her insulin, but she does eat additional snacks while snowshoeing.

Combined Insulin and Diet Changes

For snowshoeing all day, an NPH user usually eliminates her 2-unit dose of Humalog at breakfast, but she takes her usual morning dose of NPH. She always eats before working out and supplements with additional carbohydrate as needed while snowshoeing.

For vigorous snowshoeing, a pump user usually reduces the basal rate on his pump by close to 75 percent and supplements with carbohydrate as needed during the activity. He monitors his blood sugars frequently to determine when he needs to eat more.

Another Ultralente user takes no Humalog before beginning if her blood sugar is between 100 and 140 mg/dl and eats two Fig Newtons before the activity. If her blood glucose is higher than 140, she either eats less before or she takes 0.5 units of Humalog with the Fig Newtons.

Intensity, Duration, and Other Effects

An NPH user finds snowshoeing up mountains to be the most intense exercise that he does for the longest duration. He increases his food intake for the cold conditions, and he decreases his Humalog doses by 75 percent before the activity.

ICE SKATING AND IN-LINE SKATING

These activities are mainly aerobic in nature, much along the lines of walking. The gliding effect of the skates reduces some of the energy required to cover any given distance. Ice and in-line skating, if you do them at a higher skill level, may also involve powerful, quick movements such as jumping or spinning, which are more anaerobic.

The intensity and duration of skating will affect the blood sugar response to the activity. Recreational skating requires a minimal aerobic effort and uses very little blood sugar or muscle glycogen, which is similar to slow walking. Competitive skating (usually on ice) is much more intense than recreational skating and will require greater compensation. For comparable regimen changes, refer to recommendations for ice hockey in chapter 8. Skating for a longer period of time will use a greater total amount of energy and may require some minor reductions in insulin or increases in food intake, especially if you skate after a meal.

Athlete Examples

The following examples stress how the duration of skating greatly affects the necessary regimen changes. Many people can make effective adjustments with either diet or insulin changes alone.

Insulin Changes Alone

For 60 minutes of moderate in-line skating, a bedtime-only NPH user makes no preexercise adjustments to his food or insulin. However, he decreases his short-acting insulin by 2 to 3 units for all subsequent meals during the day. Another NPH user decreases

ICE SKATING AND IN-LINE SKATING

User	Insulin	Diet
NPH/Lente	• For shorter, slower-paced skating, reduce preexercise short-acting insulin doses by 20-40%. • For longer-duration, faster skating, either reduce insulin further, or increase carbohydrate intake. • For planned exercise later in the day, reduce morning NPH (if taken) by 10-30%.	• Increase carbohydrate intake by 10-20 grams at preexercise meals. • Consume 10-15 grams of carbohydrate during the activity if needed.
Insulin Pump	• Reduce basal insulin rates by 10-20% during slower, shorter bouts of skating. • For more extended efforts, reduce both the basal rate (10-20%) and boluses before exercise (20-40%).	• Increase carbohydrate intake by 10-15 grams per hour to maintain blood sugar levels for more extended efforts.
Ultralente	• Decrease short-acting insulin by 20-40% for meals before exercise. • For prolonged or faster skating, reduce insulin more, or eat an additional snack.	• Increase carbohydrate intake up to 15 grams before or during the activity. • If insulin is sufficiently reduced, a larger carbohydrate intake is usually not necessary unless skating is very prolonged.

his Humalog dose by 40 percent before the exercise, and for longer-duration skating, he may also limit the amount of NPH he takes before the exercise and add another shot of NPH later on after the exercise to compensate. A pump user reduces his preexercise meal bolus by a third for in-line skating, but he seldom needs any supplemental food during this activity.

Diet Changes Alone

For ice or in-line skating for 15 to 45 minutes at an easy to moderate pace, an NPH user eats additional carbohydrate before beginning if her blood sugar is 100 mg/dl or below, but she will not make any adjustments for a reading of 120 or above. For one to two hours of moderate in-line skating, another NPH user just snacks on additional carbohydrate as needed during the activity without making any insulin changes. A pump user finds that recreational ice skating does not have much effect on his blood sugars, so he does not adjust for this activity. For one to two hours of ice skating, an Ultralente user reduces her preactivity short-acting insulin by 1 to 2 units and supplements with carbohydrate as needed.

Combined Insulin and Diet Changes

For in-line skating of 10 miles or more, an NPH user cuts her preexercise meal Humalog by 20 to 40 percent if she plans her exercise; she eats an extra 30 grams of carbohydrate for unplanned skating. Another pump user decreases her basal rate by 50 percent about 30 minutes before beginning and keeps it reduced for the duration of the exercise (from 1.1 units per hour). She also drinks four ounces of juice if her blood sugar is below 100 mg/dl before beginning. An Ultralente user is active every day, so she makes no real adjustments to her insulin or diet for occasional in-line skating, but another Ultralente user reduces his Humalog dose by 50 percent before and doubles his carbohydrate intake during this activity.

SKATEBOARDING

This activity is mainly anaerobic, involving short bursts of intense activity such as jumping, with some aerobic use of postural muscles to maintain balance. Under these conditions, you will need minimal changes in insulin or carbohydrate intake. If you use skateboarding as a form of transportation and do it continuously, it is more aerobic in nature. Any changes in insulin or diet will depend more on the aerobic exercise component of this activity. You may need a 10 to 20 percent reduction in short-acting insulin doses before the activity combined with extra carbohydrates (0 to 15 grams per hour). Pump users may also reduce basal rates during more continuous skateboarding by 10 to 20 percent in lieu of supplementing with carbohydrate.

GOLF

This activity requires short bursts of energy for hitting, driving, and putting, which are anaerobic in nature and mainly use the phosphagen system. Walking the course is aerobic in nature and carrying golf clubs increases the workload, but driving a golf cart does not increase energy usage. The necessary regimen changes will depend mainly on the amount of aerobic exercise you do while golfing and the environmental conditions.

The amount of walking you do while golfing will have the greatest effect on blood sugars. Golfing while using a golf cart provides minimal aerobic exercise. Walking the course increases the energy expenditure significantly and requires greater regimen changes to compensate. Hotter and more humid playing conditions affect blood sugar levels more because trying to keep cool increases the body's blood glucose use. Longer playing times also require greater regimen changes.

Athlete Examples

The amount of walking you do, the temperature and humidity, and the length of golf play affect the reported regimen changes. Golfers make changes in their insulin alone, diet alone, neither, or both.

Insulin Changes Alone

A bedtime-only NPH user reduces his preexercise meal Humalog dose by 50 percent for nine holes of golf lasting two to three hours. To avoid hypoglycemia, he reduces his postexercise Humalog by 25 percent (usually 2 units) and reduce his bedtime NPH by 25 percent.

GOLF*

User	Insulin	Diet
NPH/Lente	• If walking the course, reduce short-acting insulin doses by 10-50% for any meals before or during golfing. • For afternoon golfing, reduce morning doses of NPH (if taken) by 10-30%. • Hotter conditions or longer play may require greater insulin reductions or food intake.	• Increase food intake by 5-15 grams of carbohydrate for every hour of golfing depending on the actual insulin reductions.
Insulin Pump	• If walking the course, reduce short-acting insulin doses by 10-50% for any meals before or during golfing. • Reduce basal insulin rates by 25-50% as well during the activity. • Hotter conditions or longer play may require greater insulin reductions (premeal and/or basal insulin rates) or increased carbohydrate intake.	• Eat 0-15 grams of carbohydrate per hour to compensate for the walking depending on the reductions in basal insulin.
Ultralente	• If walking the course, reduce short-acting insulin doses by 10-50% for any meals before or during golfing. • No reductions in Ultralente doses are usually necessary. • Hotter conditions or longer play may require greater reductions in short-acting insulin or larger increases in carbohydrate intake.	• Increase carbohydrate intake by 0-15 grams per hour depending on the reductions in insulin doses.

* Golfing using a golf cart will require minimal insulin and dietary changes.

For golf, a pump user usually decreases his preexercise meal bolus by 3 units, but he does not change his basal dose. If he becomes hypoglycemic during the activity, he drinks six to eight ounces of orange juice.

For 60 minutes of driving at a golfing range after dinner, an Ultralente user reduces her premeal Humalog and her Regular by 0.5 units each (a total of 1 unit less of short-acting insulins). For playing 2.5 hours of golf, another Ultralente user decreases his preexercise meal Humalog by 50 percent, but he does not change his food intake.

Diet Changes Alone

An NPH user finds that he needs to eat an extra 200 to 250 calories of carbohydrates to play nine holes of golf, but he does not adjust his insulin doses.

A pump user plays nine holes of golf for two to three hours. For this activity he eats an additional 50 grams of carbohydrate, but he does not make any insulin reductions. For four to five hours of golfing, another pump user does not make any alterations in his insulin doses because he eats extra carbohydrate as needed.

An Ultralente user eats a bit more carbohydrate while golfing and drinks a sport drink to maintain her blood sugar levels. She does not adjust her insulin dose.

Combined Insulin and Diet Changes

For golfing, an NPH user makes no changes in her insulin or food intake, but she carries supplemental carbohydrates with her on the course. Another NPH user decreases his morning NPH dose and increases his food intake during the activity if he walks while golfing. For golfing in the morning, another NPH user reduces his breakfast Humalog by 1 unit (from 5 to 4) and then eats a PowerBar by the eighth or ninth hole.

On the afternoons that a bedtime-only NPH user has golf practice, he does not make any adjustments before his activity, but he decreases his dinner Humalog by 1 unit following practice or games. He keeps juice, regular soda, glucose tablets, and candy available while golfing to treat hypoglycemia. At bedtime if his blood sugar is below 90 mg/dl, he eats an additional carbohydrate and a protein exchange with his bedtime snack.

A pump user who walks the course usually keeps his basal rate the same for golfing and balances his blood sugars with extra carbohydrates. If he eats a meal before golfing, he takes only a small Humalog dose to cover the meal and tries to exercise at least two hours after eating when the effects of Humalog start to wane.

For golfing, a pump user detaches his pump if his blood sugar is between 100 and 150 mg/dl. If his blood sugar is less than 120 mg/dl, he eats an extra 15 grams of carbohydrate before golfing.

Another pump user usually golfs 18 holes in four hours. For this activity, he reduces his basal rate to 70 percent of normal and supplements with 30 grams of carbohydrate while playing.

Another pump user usually decreases her basal rate by 25 percent if she walks the golf course. If her blood sugar is below 120 mg/dl to start, she eats 15 grams of carbohydrate before exercising, and she may eat another 15 to 30 grams of carbohydrate while playing. If she uses a golf cart, she still decreases her basal rate by 25 percent, but she does not eat any additional carbohydrates.

An Ultralente user reduces her Humalog by 1 unit before golfing and then supplements with 15 grams of carbohydrate for every hour that she plays. For 18 holes of golf while walking the course, another Ultralente user reduces his Humalog doses by 5 to 10 percent during the activity. He also supplements with carbohydrate depending on his blood sugar levels: solid sources for exercise over 90 minutes and liquids for shorter durations.

Intensity, Duration, and Other Effects

Effect of environment. If a pump user plays golf all day in the Florida heat, he may reduce his basal rate on his pump. If it is cooler when he plays, he does not normally reduce it.

Effect of duration and intensity. A pump user may set her basal rate at 0.2 units per hour (a reduction of 0.2 to 0.3 units per hour) or not adjust it at all, depending on the rate of play and the amount of walking she does.

Effect of blood sugar level. For golfing 18 holes, a pump user makes adjustments based on her starting blood sugar. For a value of less than 120 mg/dl, she reduces her basal rate during the activity from 0.7 to 0.3 units per hour while golfing and eats a banana. For blood sugar between 120 and 200, she modifies her insulin the same, but she does not eat any extra food. For blood sugar over 200 mg/dl, she reduces the basal rate to only 0.4 units per hour and does not eat a snack. She carries a diluted sport drink with her and takes three to four swallows from it at every hole. She checks her blood sugar after six to nine holes, eats a peanut butter and jelly sandwich with a piece of fruit, and takes only 75 percent of her usual mealtime bolus of Humalog with it.

TENNIS

This activity is mainly composed of short, powerful moves such as serving, returning a serve, moving into position, or hitting the ball, with extended periods of waiting in between. Due to its stop-and-start nature, it is a mix of anaerobic bursts and more aerobic activity. The intensity depends on whether the play is singles or doubles; singles play will generally require more activity by each person compared with doubles play. Both the intensity and duration of play will affect the blood sugar response and necessary regimen changes to maintain blood sugar levels.

The biggest effects on blood sugar response to tennis come from the duration of play and circulating insulin levels. Other factors can also affect the intensity of play and the blood sugar response. Longer tennis games or practices will generally have more of a glucose-reducing effect than shorter playing periods because you move more. Playing tennis early in the morning or three to four hours after the last injection of short-acting insulin when circulating insulin levels are lower will also cause more stable blood sugar levels and require fewer regimen changes. Playing singles tennis will generally require you to move more than if you play doubles. Playing singles tennis, therefore, will usually cause a greater reduction in blood sugar levels. The skill level of the players may also affect the intensity. Better players are more skilled at ball placement and may end up running less than unskilled players. High-level serving may also result in more waiting time and less active playing time.

Athlete Examples

The following examples show that you can make many different regimen changes for tennis, depending on the length and type of tennis.

Insulin Changes Alone

A Lente user who plays tennis for 60 to 90 minutes varies her insulin regimen based on the time of day she plays. If she plays in the morning, she reduces her short-acting insulin at breakfast (2 units instead of 6). If she plans to play in the afternoon, she reduces her morning dose of Lente by 2 to 4 units. For evening tennis, she reduces her dinner regular to 5 to 6 units from her usual 10 (a 40 to 50 percent reduction).

TENNIS

User	Insulin	Diet
NPH/Lente	• For shorter tennis games or practices of 30-60 minutes, reduce short-acting insulin doses 10-25% before playing depending on the intensity of play. • Reduce morning NPH by 10-20% (if taken) for playing in the afternoon. • For longer tennis games or practices lasting 1-2 hours, reduce short-acting doses by 15-40%.	• Consume an additional 15-30 grams of carbohydrate per hour for shorter-duration play, especially if insulin levels are higher (following a meal or during an NPH peak), or if insulin reductions are not made prior to playing. • Increase carbohydrate intake for longer tennis play.
Insulin Pump	• For 30-60 minutes of tennis, reduce short-acting doses of insulin by 10-25% before playing depending on the intensity of play. • Reduce basal insulin rates by 25-50% or remove the pump altogether while playing. • For longer tennis games or practices lasting 1-2 hours, reduce short-acting doses by 15-40% with similar or even greater basal rate changes.	• Consume an additional 15-30 grams of carbohydrate per hour depending on reductions in basal rates and bolus doses. • Increase carbohydrate intake even more for longer durations if insulin is not reduced.
Ultralente	• For less than an hour of tennis, reduce short-acting insulin doses by 10-25% before playing depending on the intensity of play. • Playing tennis when circulating insulin levels are lower (before a meal) may require no insulin reductions. • For longer tennis games or practices lasting 1-2 hours, reduce short-acting doses by 15-40% before playing.	• Increase carbohydrate intake by 15-30 grams per hour, especially if insulin levels are higher (within 3-4 hours following a meal) and are not reduced. • Playing tennis when circulating insulin levels are lower (before a meal) may require smaller increases in carbohydrate intake.

A pump user removes her pump for two to three hours of moderate to heavy tennis if her blood sugar is normal or low before beginning. If her blood sugar is above 200 mg/dl, she boluses 2 to 3 units of regular insulin then removes her pump to play.

Diet Changes Alone

An NPH user makes no changes in insulin dose but she eats fruit between points while playing tennis. For each hour of singles tennis, another NPH user needs to eat about 50 grams of carbo-hydrate.

An NPH user plays mixed doubles in the evening for two hours. For this activity she eats a higher-protein, lower-carbohydrate snack before beginning and delays taking her dinnertime NPH until after playing when she eats dinner. Another NPH user eats 15 to 30 grams of extra carbohydrates before playing two hours of doubles tennis, depending on her blood sugar level, and a minimum of 15 grams of carbohydrate afterward, regardless of her blood sugars.

For doubles, a pump user does not make any alterations in his insulin doses. He prefers to eat extra carbohydrate before and during the activity as needed.

For 30 to 60 minutes of tennis, an Ultralente user eats one piece of fruit 30 minutes before beginning but makes no adjustments to his insulin dose. Another Ultralente user does not adjust his insulin for tennis (90 minutes to two hours), but he does drink a sport drink and juice mixture on the court while playing and tests his blood sugar frequently.

Combined Insulin and Diet Changes

An NPH user decreases her preexercise meal regular by 1 to 3 units and then drinks eight to 16 ounces of juice as needed before playing tennis. Another NPH user plays doubles tennis for two or more hours at a time. He typically reduces his preexercise meal Humalog by 10 to 40 percent (he usually takes 6 to 10 units for each meal) and keeps a glucose solution nearby to drink as needed.

For 30 minutes of tennis, a pump user disconnects his pump. For longer bouts, he only decreases the basal rate to 30 to 50 percent of normal during the activity. If necessary, he takes 15 to 20 grams of glucose before 30 minutes of exercise. For one to two hours of tennis, another pump user decreases her basal rate from 0.3 to 0.4 units per hour to 0.1 to 0.2 units and increases her food intake. For singles tennis lasting 90 minutes to two hours, another pump user suspends his pump while playing and additionally supplements with 45 to 75 grams of carbohydrates per exercise session. Another pump user checks her blood sugar before playing and tries to start with her blood sugar at 150 to 200 mg/dl. If she plays for over two hours, she decreases her basal pump rate by 50 percent and uses glucose tablets to correct hypoglycemia.

An Ultralente user usually plays 30 minutes to two hours of tennis at a time. For this activity, she takes 1 unit less of Humalog for the meal before playing. If it has been more than an hour since her last meal, she drinks some milk and eats a protein and carbohydrate snack before playing. She also drinks a carbohydrate beverage and water for every 30 minutes of tennis.

INDOOR RACKET SPORTS: RACQUETBALL, HANDBALL, SQUASH, AND BADMINTON

Racket sports involve quick, powerful moves such as hitting or throwing the ball and moving into position. These activities are mostly anaerobic in nature. Primarily the intensity and length of play as well as skill level determine the insulin and diet changes for these activities.

The duration of play and the circulating insulin levels during these indoor racket activities have the biggest effects on blood sugar response. Various factors can also affect the intensity of play. Longer playing periods will generally have more of a glucose-reducing effect than shorter ones because more total activity is done. Exercising when circulating insulin levels are lower (early in the morning or three to four hours after the last injection of short-acting insulin) also generally allows for more stable blood sugar levels with fewer regimen changes. The skill level of the players may also affect the intensity. Better players are more skilled at ball placement and may end up running less than unskilled players. Well-placed, point-winning serves may also result in more waiting time and less active playing time.

Athlete Examples

These examples show that court sports are intense enough to require some regimen changes to prevent hypoglycemia. More prolonged play has more of an aerobic effect as well.

RACKET SPORTS: RACQUETBALL, HANDBALL, SQUASH, BADMINTON

User	Insulin	Diet
NPH/Lente	• For shorter durations (30-60 minutes), reduce short-acting insulin doses by 10-25% before playing. • Reduce morning NPH doses by a similar amount (if taken) for playing in the afternoon, or eat an additional snack before playing. • For longer games lasting 1-2 hours, reduce short-acting doses by 15-40%.	• Consume 15-30 grams of carbohydrate per hour as well, especially if insulin levels are higher (following a meal or during an NPH peak), or if you make minimal reductions in insulin before playing. • Eat additional carbohydrate for longer games as needed.
Insulin Pump	• For shorter durations (30-60 minutes), reduce short-acting insulin doses by 10-25% before playing. • Reduce basal insulin rates by 25-50%, or remove the pump altogether during the activity. • For longer games lasting 1-2 hours, reduce short-acting doses by 15-40% before exercise, and reduce basal rates by 50-75% during play.	• Consume an additional 15-30 grams of carbohydrate per hour depending on the actual reductions in basal insulin rates and bolus doses. • Eat additional carbohydrate for longer games as needed, depending on insulin reductions.
Ultralente	• For shorter durations (30-60 minutes), reduce short-acting insulin doses by 10-25% before playing, depending on the intensity of play. • If playing when circulating insulin levels are lower (before a meal), make minimal insulin reductions and increases in carbohydrate intake. • For longer games lasting 1-2 hours, reduce short-acting doses by 15-40% before playing.	• For shorter durations, eat an additional 15-30 grams of carbohydrate per hour, especially if insulin levels are higher (within 3-4 hours following a meal). • For longer games, increase carbohydrate intake.

Insulin Changes Alone

An NPH user reduces his short-acting insulin by 2 units before playing one to two hours of squash. He does not usually need to make any dietary adjustments.

Diet Changes Alone

For playing squash, an NPH user tests his blood sugar, snacks, plays, and then tests his blood sugar again. He does not make any adjustments to his Humalog dose before playing.

For squash, a pump user makes dietary adjustments based on his blood sugar readings before beginning, but he does not adjust his basal rate or his boluses. Another pump user increases the carbohydrates in a meal before 60 minutes of hard racquetball, but he does not adjust his basal dose on his pump for this activity.

Combined Insulin and Diet Changes

An NPH user decreases his regular insulin by 10 to 20 percent or increases his food intake, depending on actual racquetball playing time. For racquetball, another NPH user may take 2 to 3 units less of Regular insulin or eat up to 500 calories' worth of additional snacks to maintain his blood sugar during the activity.

For playing racquetball, a pump user suspends his pump if his blood sugar is between 100 and 150 mg/dl. If his blood sugar is less than 120, he eats an extra 15 grams of carbohydrate before this activity. Another pump user suspends his pump for up to two hours of playing. He tests his blood sugar and adjusts with carbohydrates every 30 minutes as needed.

An Ultralente user decreases her regular insulin before a game and drinks sport drinks during the breaks for 40 to 60 minutes of racquetball. If involved in a tournament for the weekend, she decreases her Ultralente dose by 30 to 40 percent for those days. At times, she uses no regular insulin when she plays more than five games in a day. She tests her blood sugar frequently during these tournaments to make insulin and food adjustments.

Intensity, Duration, and Other Effects

Effect of time of day. For intense racquetball lasting 45 to 90 minutes, an NPH user varies his insulin and food based on the time of day he plays. If he plays before a meal, he tries to eat a bit, exercise, then test his blood sugar and dose according to his blood sugar and his planned food. If he plays after a meal, he usually cuts back on his NPH dose by 1 unit and waits three to four hours to play because he finds it difficult to exercise until most of his Regular insulin is gone from his system. An Ultralente user usually plays racquetball intensely for 60 minutes in the early morning. For this activity, he does not make any adjustments to his food or insulin, but he does wait to take his insulin injection until after he is finished.

DANCE: BALLET, MODERN, SOCIAL, AND BALLROOM

These activities can be a combination of aerobic and anaerobic activities, depending on the intensity and duration of the dance movements. Ballet requires power moves, such as jumping, and sustained muscular contractions when holding dance positions. Other types of dance are generally more aerobic in nature but they are usually low-level activities. Insulin or diet changes will depend on the intensity and duration of the particular form of dance.

The intensity and duration of dancing will have the biggest effects on blood sugar responses. Social or recreational dance may not exert much of a glucose-reducing effect. More intense forms of dance such as ballet classes can be much more rigorous and require greater changes in insulin or food intake.

Athlete Examples

These people choose to make changes primarily in their diet, and the actual adjustment depends on the type of dance they do.

Diet Changes Alone

For social dance, an NPH user makes no adjustments in her insulin or food intake. For dancing in the late evenings, another NPH user finds that she may need a larger bedtime snack. She does not adjust her insulin doses, though. For a 75-minute ballet class, an Ultralente user usually has something light to eat or drink, such as a café latte, before teaching the class. If her blood sugar is more than 250, she takes 1 unit of Humalog before class. For Irish step dance, another Ultralente user will eat extra carbohydrates as needed without adjusting her insulin doses.

Combined Insulin and Diet Changes

For three to four hours of country-western dance, a pump user generally eats more snacks or an extra meal and decreases her boluses slightly depending on the duration and intensity of the activity.

For professional ballet, an NPH user does not take any short-acting insulin before performing. She checks her blood sugar levels

DANCE: BALLET, MODERN, SOCIAL, BALLROOM

User	Insulin	Diet
NPH/Lente	• Make minimal changes in insulin and diet for most social or recreational dance. • Reduce short-acting insulin by 10-20% for dancing after a meal or during peak insulin times. • For more intense or prolonged dancing such as ballet classes, reduce insulin by 20-40% unless circulating insulin levels are low during the activity (3-4 hours after the last injection of short-acting insulin).	• Increase carbohydrate intake by 0-15 grams per hour for most social or recreational dance. • Increase carbohydrate intake by 10-30 grams per hour for prolonged or intense dancing such as ballet.
Insulin Pump	• Reduce basal insulin rates by 0-20% during the activity done at a low level (social or recreational dance). • If the activity follows a meal, reduce premeal boluses by 10-20%. • For more intense or prolonged dancing, reduce basal rates and boluses by 20-40% before and/or during the activity.	• Increase carbohydrate intake by 0-15 grams per hour during the activity. • Eat an additional 10-30 grams of carbohydrate per hour for intense or prolonged dancing.
Ultralente	• Make few changes in insulin and diet for most social or recreational dance, especially if done when circulating insulin levels are low. • For dancing after a meal, reduce short-acting insulin by 10-20%. • For more intense or prolonged dance or ballet classes, reduce short-acting insulin by 20-40%.	• Increase carbohydrate intake by 0-15 grams per hour for dancing after a meal. • Increase carbohydrate intake by 10-30 grams per hour for more prolonged or intense dance.

frequently (at times before, during, and after the activity) and eats carbohydrate to maintain her blood sugar levels on the high side. She finds that the extreme amount of physical activity she does requires much lower insulin doses overall, and she has to eat additional snacks following particularly strenuous workouts or performances to prevent later-onset hypoglycemia.

BOWLING

This activity involves very short bursts of activity (swinging and releasing the ball) and is very reliant on the quick energy (phosphagen) system. The majority of the time, little activity is being done in between bowls. Consequently, the total energy expended while bowling is minimal, its effect on blood sugar is usually insignificant, and few regimen changes are likely to be needed with any diabetes regimen. However, for prolonged participation (2 to 3 hours) or more competitive bowling, a small increase in food intake may be needed (5 to 10 grams of carbohydrate), especially if play is occurring during peak insulin times in NPH or Lente users. For insulin pump users, basal insulin rates may be decreased a small amount (10 to 20 percent) during prolonged bowling.

YARD WORK

This activity is both anaerobic and aerobic in nature. It requires using muscles to maintain balance (usually postural muscles that are more aerobic in nature) and other muscles for repetitious motions (raking, mowing, weeding, and other activities). The anaerobic component is elicited by the quick recruitment of additional muscles to perform more forceful activities (carrying waste bags, digging a hole, hoeing, etc.). A more prolonged effort will necessitate greater regimen changes. More intense work (like chopping wood or shoveling) can also cause a greater reduction in blood sugar levels, especially when the activity is more prolonged.

Athlete Examples

The following examples show that yard work can be accounted for by any sort of regimen change, depending on its intensity and duration.

Insulin Changes Alone

A pump user finds that for heavy housework and yard work, she needs to decrease her boluses of Humalog prior to the activity by 1 to 2 units. For heavy gardening, another pump user reduces the basal rate on her pump from 0.4 to 0.5 units per hour down to 0.1 to 0.2 units during the activity, depending on the intensity.

Diet Changes Alone

An Ultralente user counts regular gardening in one-hour bouts as exercise. She usually eats 10 to 20 grams of extra carbohydrate for this activity unless it replaces one of her usual activities.

Combined Insulin and Diet Changes

An NPH user finds that for 2 to 3 hours of high-intensity yard work, he does not take his normal dose of Regular insulin, and he has to eat additional carbohydrate every 90 to 120 minutes to avoid low blood sugars. For strenuous or prolonged yard work, a pump user finds that she needs to eat an additional snack if she does not reduce her basal rate by 25 to 50 percent during the activity. For heavy raking, another pump user suspends her pump during the activity and adds extra carbohydrate as needed. An Ultralente user finds that for wood cutting (which he considers heavy exercise), he has to reduce his preexercise meal humalog by 50 percent (or at least two units) and eat an apple every 90 minutes to prevent low blood sugars.

EXERCISE IN ENVIRONMENTAL EXTREMES: HEAT, HUMIDITY, COLD, AND ALTITUDE

Aerobic or prolonged activities in environmental extremes will increase the overall energy used by increasing metabolic rate; the body's reliance on carbohydrate energy sources is also usually enhanced. Exercise in a warm or hot environment may speed the rate of insulin absorption from an injection site as well because blood flow to the skin is increased even more than usual for sweating and cooling purposes. Many people have noticed significant effects on blood sugar while exercising in all of these more extreme environments. You will need to make regimen changes to compensate for the greater use of both blood glucose and muscle glycogen under these conditions.

The duration of exercise in environmental extremes will determine its additional effect on blood sugar levels. The more prolonged the activity, the greater the effect the environment has to stimulate greater blood glucose and muscle glycogen use. The degree of extremity of the environment will also have an effect. Hot and humid conditions increase energy expenditure more than heat alone; wind chill exacerbates the effects of coldness, and higher altitudes affect the blood sugar response more than lower elevations.

Combined Insulin and Diet Changes

All people can use a combination of insulin and diet changes to compensate for exercise in extreme environmental conditions. The greater use of blood glucose and muscle glycogen for exercise in these conditions will require a reduction in insulin, increase in carbohydrate intake, or both to effectively maintain blood sugar levels during the activity. Any insulin reductions and carbohydrate supplementation beyond what is normally expected for the exercise itself would be greater as well. The duration of exercise and the environmental conditions determine the necessary changes.

Athlete Examples

These examples include regimen changes for golfing in the heat, skiing in the cold at altitude, and hiking in the mountains at altitude, among other activities.

Insulin Changes Alone

For golfing all day in the Florida heat and humidity, a pump user may reduce the basal rate on his pump, although he does not usually do so for golfing in cooler weather. A pump user finds that she has to cut back on her Regular insulin dose by 50 percent when she skis at altitude and in the cold because that environment causes her blood sugars to drop severely. Another pump user finds that exercising at altitude increases her workload, especially if running up a mountain. For running at higher altitudes, she decreases the basal rate on her pump to 0.1 or 0.2 units per hour from her usual 0.5. This adjustment is even greater than for running at her usual altitude of 8,000 feet.

Diet Changes Alone

A pump user finds that exercising in the heat causes her blood sugar to drop more rapidly, so she needs to drink carbohydrate fluids every 30 minutes and monitor her blood sugar more frequently. She finds she often gets hypoglycemic during the night if she exercises all day in hot and humid weather. Another pump user has to eat an extra glucose tablet every 15 minutes and drink more water while exercising in the heat. For exercise in the cold, an Ultralente user increases his dietary fat intake as well as his carbohydrate intake during the activity.

Combined Insulin and Diet Changes

Effect of a hot, humid environment. For exercise in the heat, an NPH user decreases her preexercise meal regular by 1 to 3 units and then drinks eight to 16 ounces of juice before beginning her exercise. She also drinks a lot of extra water during and after the activity. A pump user finds that playing tennis in a hot environment causes a dramatic drop in his blood sugar. He usually suspends his pump and drinks water before and a sport drink while playing in the evening. An Ultralente user finds that running or cycling in the heat reduces his blood sugar levels an additional 20 to 25 percent more than during normal environmental conditions. He judges the effect of the heat based on the ambient temperature and relative humidity. For hotter and more humid conditions, he has to make greater adjustments in his insulin and/or carbohydrate intake to compensate for his body's greater use of blood sugar under those conditions.

Effect of altitude and a cold environment. During a backpacking trip when she hiked for six to eight hours a day at altitude, an NPH user decreased her total intake of insulin by 60 percent and doubled her food intake. For mountain climbing in the cold at altitude, another NPH user reduces his short-acting insulin during the activity and eats more food including chocolate bars.

A pump user finds that hiking over 14,000 feet up Mt. Shasta requires major alterations in her insulin doses and carbohydrate intake. During the activity, she most often decreases her basal rate by 50 percent (from 0.8 units per hour to 0.4), checks her blood sugar every 30 to 60 minutes, and takes glucose gels (about 30 grams of carbohydrate) as needed and eats additional carbohydrate snacks.

For a three-week backpacking trip in the Himalayas at altitudes over 15,000 feet, an Ultralente user took even less insulin than he usually does for backpacking. He reduced his overall insulin by more than 50 percent, did not take his usual basal Ultralente dose, and took multiple small doses of Regular insulin (he usually takes

Humalog) on the trail in accordance with frequent blood sugar tests and snacking along the trail. One day in the mountains at 20,000 feet, he only took 6 units of insulin all day compared with his usual dose of about 50 units, and he had perfect blood sugars.

From this chapter you can see that diabetes does not keep individuals from participating in every conceivable sport and recreational physical activity. Although not profiled in this chapter because it is so unusual, one individual even returned a survey describing his regimen changes for "dog mushing" in Alaska! So go ahead and learn how to water ski, hike up a mountain, ski down the Alps, become certified to scuba dive, in-line skate in the park, and just have fun being physically active despite your diabetes!

appendix A

DIABETIC ATHLETES AND SPORT ORGANIZATIONS

American College of Sports Medicine
Street address: 401 W. Michigan St., Indianapolis, IN 46202-3233
Mailing Address: P.O. Box 1440, Indianapolis, IN 46202-1440
Phone: 317-637-9200
Fax: 317-634-7817
Web site: **www.acsm.org**

American Diabetes Association
Address: 1660 Duke Street
Alexandria, VA 22314
Phone: 703-549-1500 or 800-342-2383
Fax: 703-549-1715
E-mail: customerservice@diabetes.org
Web site: **www.diabetes.org**

International Diabetic Athletes Association
Address: 1647-B West Bethany Home Road
Phoenix, AZ 85015
Phone: 602-433-2113 or 800-898-IDAA
Fax: 602-433-9331
E-mail: idaa@diabetes-exercise.org
Web site: **www.diabetes-exercise.org**

Juvenile Diabetes Foundation
Address: 120 Wall Street, 19th Floor
New York, NY 10005
Phone: 212-785-9500 or 800-533-2873
Fax: 212-785-9595
E-mail: info@jdfcure.org
Web site: **www.jdfcure.org**

appendix B

SPORT AND NUTRITION WEB SITES OF INTEREST

*The following Web sites were available at the time of publication.

www.acefitness.org

This site is the official Web site of the American Council on Exercise, a non-profit organization targeting personal fitness trainers. It offers some fitness facts applicable to all people.

www.gssiweb.com

This site is the official Web site of the Gatorade Sports Science Institute. The site was created by the Gatorade Company, which is very proactive in its research in exercise science and fitness-related issues. It contains links to publications on sports medicine, sport nutrition, and exercise science under "Reference Library."

www.medscape.com

This site is a free Internet medical site. On this site you can search for any medically related topic or patient information published in journals or newspapers.

www.nal.usda.gov/fnic/foodcomp

This site provides access to USDA food nutrient data. On this site you can find out the nutritional content of any food or drink including calories, macronutrients, vitamins, and minerals.

www.navigator.tufts.edu

This site provides a rating guide to various nutrition websites. Click on the "General Nutrition" section to access these ratings and links.

www.olympic-usa.org

This site is the official Web site of the United States Olympic Committee. It contains such items as "Sports A to Z," which you can use to look up almost any sport and recap current events as well as rules of the sport. A section titled "The Games" contains information on past, current, and future Olympic Games.

www.sfu.ca/~jfremont/nutritionlinks.html

This site provides links to other nutrition-oriented Web sites including international, Canadian, U.S. government, and American university nutrition sites as well as information on exercise physiology, sports, medical, and vegetarian links.

www.sportsquest.com

This site allows you to search a wide variety of different sports and activities and provides a list of links for additional information. It also provides access to SportDiscus, an online database for sports and fitness research articles, which can be obtained for a fee.

www.sportsci.org

This site contains *SportScience*, a peer-reviewed site for sport research. New issues are posted quarterly containing up-to-date information and links to related topics.

www.thedietchannel.com

This site provides many links to articles in weight loss, sport nutrition and supplements, vitamins, minerals, food and diet analysis tools, ideal body weight and body fat calculators, and healthy living information.

Diabetic Athlete Activity Questionnaire

Name_____ Age_____ Sex_____

Years with diabetes_____ Last hemoglobin A_{1C}%_____ Date_____

Address_____
_____

Phone _____ Fax _____

E-mail _____Today's Date _____

Do you wish to remain anonymous in my publication?   YES   NO   (circle one)

Normal insulin/medication regimen

    Type of insulin(s) /diabetes medications_____

    Usual dosage and times taken_____

    Pump user? YES   NO   (circle one)

Normal exercise routine:

    Number of days a week _____

    Activities _____

    Intensity (if monitored) _____

    Duration _____

Normal dietary patterns:

    Do you follow any special diet? YES   NO   (circle one)

    Do you count carbohydrates?   YES   NO

    Do you monitor or restrict your fat intake?   YES   NO

    Do you follow ADA or other guidelines for diet?   YES   NO

    Describe your usual diet_____
    _____

Normal alterations in regimen for exercise:

    Type of exercise_____

    Insulin or medication adjustments_____

    Dietary adjustments _____

    Other_____

For the following sports and activities, please fully describe the level of involvement for any that you currently participate in or have participated in. Describe your average daily routine for that particular activity including intensity, frequency, and duration. Include any variations in your level of involvement for the activity (e.g., do you have long practices on most days, with a short, intense competition once a week?). Most importantly, describe in detail any adjustments that you make or have made in your insulin or medication regimen or dietary intake to maintain blood glucose levels in a normal or near-normal range during and following the activity. If any activity that you engage in is not on the list, add it. Feel free to use any of the space provided, or attach additional sheets.

Aerobic dance/step aerobics/hip-hop

Backpacking/hiking

Baseball/softball/t-ball

Basketball

Bowling

Boxing/kickboxing

Canoeing/kayaking

Cross country/track and field

Cross-country skiing/NordicTrack

Cycling/stationary cycling/mountain biking

Dance: ballet/modern/social/ballroom

Downhill skiing/snowboarding

Exercise in heat/cold/altitude

Field hockey

Football

Golf

Gymnastics

Hockey

Horseback riding

Jetskiing

Karate/judo/martial arts

Lacrosse

Marathons

Racquetball/handball

Rock climbing

Rowing: crew/rowing machine

Running/jogging

Sailing

Scuba/snorkeling

Skateboarding

Skating: ice/in-line/roller

Skydiving

Snowshoeing

Snowmobiling

Soccer

Stair climber/StairMaster

Swimming

Surfing

Tennis

Triathlons

Ultraendurance events

Volleyball/sand volleyball

Walking/racewalking

Waterskiing

Water aerobics

Weight training/circuit training

Windsurfing

Wrestling

Other sport or activity

For the following general guidelines for exercise and type 1 diabetes from *Clinical Practice Recommendations 2000* from the American Diabetes Association, please indicate the extent that you follow the guideline by circling the most applicable number. Also, give specific details about your personal modifications whenever possible. (It is my hope to further revise these guidelines with your input so that they are also more usable for people with type 1 diabetes and other insulin users.)

> 1 = I follow this guideline exactly
>
> 2 = I follow this guideline most of the time
>
> 3 = I follow this guideline sometimes
>
> 4 = I follow this guideline very infrequently
>
> 5 = I follow this guideline almost never

1. Metabolic control before exercise

A. Avoid exercising if fasting glucose levels are >250 mg/dl and ketosis is present, and use caution if glucose levels are >300 mg/dl and no ketosis is present.

   1   2   3   4   5

Modifications _____

B. Ingest added carbohydrate if glucose levels are <100 mg/dl.

   1   2   3   4   5

Modifications _____

2. Blood glucose monitoring before and after exercise

A. Identify when changes in insulin or food intake are necessary.

   1   2   3   4   5

Modifications _____

B. Learn the glycemic response to different exercise conditions.

   1   2   3   4   5

Modifications _____

3. Food intake

A. Consume added carbohydrate as needed to avoid hypoglycemia.

   1   2   3   4   5

Modifications _____

B. Carbohydrate-based foods should be readily available during and after exercise.

   1   2   3   4   5

Modifications _____

Additional recommendations from old guidelines for prolonged and strenuous exercise

A. Ingest 15 to 30 grams of carbohydrate for every 30 minutes of intense exercise.

   1   2   3   4   5

Modifications _____

B. Consume a snack of carbohydrate soon after exercising.

   1   2   3   4   5

Modifications _____

C. Adjust the insulin dose.

  1. Intermediate-acting insulin—decrease the dose by 30 to 35 percent on the day of exercise.

   1   2   3   4   5

   Modifications _____

  2. Intermediate- and short-acting insulin—omit the dose if it normally precedes exercise.

   1   2   3   4   5

   Modifications _____

  3. Multiple doses of short-acting insulin—reduce the dose before exercise by 30 percent and supplement with carbohydrate intake.

   1   2   3   4   5

   Modifications _____

  4. Continuous subcutaneous insulin infusion—eliminate mealtime bolus or insulin increment that precedes or follows exercise.

   1   2   3   4   5

   Modifications _____

D. Avoid exercising for 1 hour those muscles that short-acting insulin was injected into.

   1   2   3   4   5

Modifications _____

E. Avoid exercising in the late evening.

   1   2   3   4   5

Modifications _____

Note: If you would like your responses to be included in the next edition of this book, please photocopy the preceding pages and send your completed copy of the Diabetic Athlete Activity Questionnaire to the following address:

Sheri Colberg, PhD
Department of Exercise Science, PE, and Recreation (ESPER)
Old Dominion University
Norfolk, Virginia 23529-0196

If you would prefer, I can also e-mail the questionnaire to you as an attachment in either Microsoft Word or WordPerfect. I can be reached at the following address:

scolberg@odu.edu

Thank you for your interest and participation!

suggested readings

American College of Sports Medicine. 2000. *ACSM's Guidelines for Exercise Testing and Prescription*, 6th Ed. Baltimore, MD: Lippincott, Williams & Wilkins.

American Diabetes Association. 1994. *The Fitness Book.* Alexandria, VA: American Diabetes Association.

Berg, K.E. 1986. *Diabetic's Guide to Health and Fitness.* Champaign, IL: Leisure Press.

Brooks, G.A., T. Fahey, T. White, and K. Baldwin. 2000. *Exercise Physiology: Human Bioenergetics and Its Applications*, 3rd Ed. Mountain View, CA: Mayfield Publishing Company.

Campaigne, B., and R. Lampman. 1994. *Exercise in the Clinical Management of Diabetes.* Champaign, IL: Human Kinetics.

Devlin, J., and N. Ruderman, Eds. 1995. *The Health Professional's Guide to Diabetes and Exercise.* Alexandria, VA: American Diabetes Association.

Gordon, N. 1993. *Diabetes: Your Complete Exercise Guide.* Champaign, IL: Human Kinetics.

Graham, C., J. Biermann, and B. Toohey. 1995. *The Diabetes Sports and Exercise Book.* Los Angeles, CA: Lowell House.

McArdle, W.D., F.I. Katch, and V.L. Katch. 1999. *Essentials of Exercise Physiology.* Baltimore, MD: Lippincott, Williams & Wilkins.

Williams, M.H. 1999. *Nutrition for Health, Fitness, and Sport*, 5th Ed. Boston, MA: McGraw-Hill.

Williams, M.H. 1998. *The Ergogenics Edge: Pushing the Limits of Sports Performance.* Champaign, IL: Human Kinetics.

references

Chapter 1

American College of Sports Medicine. 2000. *ACSM's Guidelines for Exercise Testing and Prescription,* 6th ed. Baltimore, MD: Lippincott, Williams & Wilkins.

Chapter 2

Bak, J., U. Jacobsen, F. Jorgensen, and O. Pedersen. 1989. Insulin receptor function and glycogen synthase activity in skeletal muscle biopsies from patients with insulin-dependent diabetes mellitus: Effects of physical training. *Journal of Clinical Endocrinology and Metabolism* 69:158-164.

Colberg, S.R., J.M. Hagberg, S.D. McCole, J.M. Zmuda, P.D. Thompson, and D.E. Kelley. 1996. Utilization of glycogen but not plasma glucose is reduced in individuals with NIDDM during mild-intensity exercise. *Journal of Applied Physiology* 81:2027-2033.

Coyle, E., A. Coggan, M. Hemmert, and J. Ivy. 1986. Muscle glycogen utilization during prolonged strenuous exercise when fed carbohydrates. *Journal of Applied Physiology* 61:165-172.

Hirsch, I.B., J.C. Marker, J. Smith, R. Spina, C.A. Parvin, J.O. Holloszy, and P.E. Cryer. 1991. Insulin and glucagon in the prevention of hypoglycemia during exercise in humans. *American Journal of Physiology* 260:E695-E704.

Kjaer, M., C. Hollenbeck, B. Frey-Hewitt, H. Galbo, W. Haskell, and G. Reaven. 1990. Glucoregulation and hormonal responses to maximal exercise in non-insulin-dependent diabetes. *Journal of Applied Physiology* 68:2067-2074.

Mitchell, T.H., G. Abraham, A. Schiffrin, L.A. Leiter, and E.B. Marliss. 1988. Hyperglycemia after intense exercise in IDDM subjects during continuous subcutaneous insulin infusion. *Diabetes Care* 11:311-317.

Price, T.B., D.L. Rothman, R. Taylor, M.J. Avison, G.I. Shulman, and R.G. Shulman. 1994. Human muscle glycogen resynthesis after exercise: Insulin-dependent and -independent phases. *Journal of Applied Physiology* 76:104-111.

Raguso, C.A., A.R. Coggan, A. Gastaldelli, L.S. Sidossis, E.J. Bastyr, 3rd, and R.R. Wolfe. 1995. Lipid and carbohydrate metabolism in IDDM during moderate and intense exercise. *Diabetes* 44:1066-1074.

Richter, E., L. Turcotte, P. Hespel, and B. Kiens. 1992. Metabolic responses to exercise: Effects of endurance training and implications for diabetes. *Diabetes Care* 15:1767-1776.

Sigal, R.J., C. Purdon, S.J. Fisher, J.B. Halter, M. Vranic, and E.B. Marliss. 1994. Hyperinsulinemia prevents prolonged hyperglycemia after intense exercise in insulin-dependent diabetic subjects. *Journal of Clinical Endocrinology and Metabolism* 79:1049-1057.

Soo, K., S.M. Furler, K. Samaras, A.B. Jenkins, L.V. Campbell, and D.J. Chisholm. 1996. Glycemic responses to exercise in IDDM after simple and complex carbohydrate supplementation. *Diabetes Care* 19:575-579.

Tuominen, J., P. Ebeling, H. Vuorinen-Markkola, and V. Koivisto. 1997. Post-marathon paradox in IDDM: Unchanged insulin sensitivity in spite of glycogen depletion. *Diabetic Medicine* 14:301-308.

Zander, E., W. Bruns, P. Wulfert, W. Besch, D. Lubs, R. Chlup, and B. Schulz. 1983. Muscular exercise in type 1-diabetics: I. Different metabolic reactions during heavy muscular work is dependent on actual insulin availability. *Experimental and Clinical Endocrinology* 82:78-90.

Zander, E., B. Schulz, R. Chlup, P. Woltansky, and D. Lubs. 1985. Muscular exercise in type 1-diabetics: II. Hormonal and metabolic responses to moderate exercise. *Experimental and Clinical Endocrinology* 85:95-104.

Chapter 3

Feinglos, M. and M. Bethel. 1999. Oral agent therapy in the treatment of type 2 diabetes. *Diabetes Care* 22 (Suppl. 3):C61-C64.

Ratner, R.E., I.B. Hirsch, J.L. Neifing, S.K. Garg, T.E. Mecca, and C.A. Wilson. 2000. Less hypoglycemia with insulin Glargine in intensive insulin therapy for type 1 diabetes. *Diabets Care* 23(5): 639-643.

Ruegemer, J.J., R.W. Squires, H.M. March, M.W. Haymond, P.E. Cryer, R.A. Rizza, and J.M. Miles. 1990. Differences between prebreakfast and late afternoon glycemic responses to exercise in IDDM patients. *Diabetes Care* 13:104-110.

Sonnenberg, G., F. Kemmer, and M. Berger. 1990. Exercise in type 1 (insulin-dependent) diabetic patients treated with continuous subcutaneous insulin infusion: Prevention of exercise induce hypoglycemia. *Diabetologia* 33:696-703.

Chapter 4

Bahrke, M.S., and W.P. Morgan. 1994. Evaluation of the ergogenic properties of ginseng. *Sports Medicine* 18:229-248.

Bursell, S.-E., A.C. Clermont, L.P. Aiello, L.M. Aiello, D.K. Schlossman, E.P. Feener, L. Laffel, and G.L. King. 1999. High-dose vitamin E supplementation normalizes retinal blood flow and creatinine clearance in patients with type 1 diabetes. *Diabetes Care* 22:1245-1251.

Clarkson, P.M. 1996. Nutrition for improved sports performance: Current issues on ergogenic aids. *Sports Medicine* 21:293-401.

Clarkson, P.M., and E.M. Haymes. 1994. Trace mineral requirements for athletes. *International Journal of Sport Nutrition* 4:104-119.

Costill, D.L., and M. Hargreaves. 1992. Carbohydrate nutrition and fatigue. *Sports Medicine* 13:86-92.

Coyle, E.F. 1994. Fluid and carbohydrate replacement during exercise: How much and why? *Sports Science Exchange* 7(3):1-6.

Faure, P., P.Y. Benhamou, A. Perard, S. Halimi, and A.M. Roussel. 1995. Lipid peroxidation in insulin-dependent diabetic patients with early retina degenerative lesions: Effects of an oral zinc supplementation. *European Journal of Clinical Nutrition* 49:282-288.

Faure, P., A. Roussel, C. Coudray, M.J. Richard, S. Halimi, and A. Favier. 1992. Zinc and insulin sensitivity. *Biological Trace Element Research* 32:305-310.

Goldfarb, A. 1993. Antioxidants: Role of supplementation to prevent exercise-induced oxidative stress. *Medicine and Science in Sports and Exercise* 25:232-236.

Kanter, M.M. 1994. Free radicals, exercise, and antioxidant supplementation. *International Journal of Sport Nutrition* 4:205-220.

Lefavi, R.G., R.A. Anderson, R.E. Keith, G.D. Wilson, J.L. McMillan, and M.H. Stone. 1992. Efficacy of chromium supplementation in athletes: Emphasis on anabolism. *International Journal of Sport Nutrition* 2:111-112.

Legwold, G. 1994. Hydration breakthrough! A sponge called glycerol boosts endurance by super-loading your body with water. *Bicycling* 35(7):72-74.

Lemon, P.W. 1995. Do athletes need more dietary protein and amino acids? *International Journal of Sport Nutrition* 5:S39-S51.

Maughan, R.J. 1995. Creatine supplementation and exercise performance. *International Journal of Sport Nutrition* 5:94-101.

McDonald, R., and C.L. Keen. 1988. Iron, zinc, and magnesium nutrition and athletic performance. *Sports Medicine* 5:171-184.

Nehlig, A. and G. Debry. 1994. Caffeine and sport activity: A review. *International Journal of Sport Nutrition* 15:215-223.

Spriet, L. 1995. Caffeine and performance. *International Journal of Sport Nutrition* 5:S84-S99.

Vuksan, V., J.L. Sievenpiper, V.Y. Koo, T. Francis, U. Beljan-Zdravkovic, Z. Xu, and E. Vidgen. 2000. American ginseng (*Panax quinquefolius* L.) reduces postprandial glycemia in nondiabetic subjects and subjects with type 2 diabetes mellitus. *Archives of Internal Medicine* 160: 1009-1013.

Williams, M.H. 1999. *Nutrition for Health, Fitness, and Sport,* 5th Ed. Boston, MA: McGraw-Hill.

Williams, M.H. 1998. *The Erogenics Edge: Pushing the Limits of Sports Performance.* Champaign, IL: Human Kinetics.

Williams, M.H. 1989. Vitamin supplementation and athletic performance. *International Journal of Vitamin and Nutrition Research* 30 (Suppl.):163-191.

Chapter 5

American Diabetes Association. 2000. Diabetes mellitus and exercise. *Diabetes Care* 23 (Suppl. 1):S50-S54.

Colberg, S.R. 2000. Use of clinical practice recommendation for exercise by individuals with type 1 diabetes. *The Diabetes Educator* 26(2):122-126.

Ivy, J.L., S.L. Katz, C.L. Cutler, W.M. Sherman, and E.F. Coyle. 1988. Muscle glycogen synthesis after exercise: Effect of time of carbohydrate ingestion. *Journal of Applied Physiology* 64:1480-1485.

MacDonald, M.J. 1987. Post-exercise late-onset hypoglycemia in insulin-dependent diabetic patients. *Diabetes Care* 10:584-588.

Chapter 6

Houmard, J.A., N.J. Bruno, R.K. Bruner, M.R. McCammon, and R.G. Israel. 1993. Effects of exercise training on the chemical composition of plasma LDL. *Atherosclerosis and Thrombosis* 14:325-330.

index

*The letters *t* and *f* indicate tables and figures.

A

Acarbose 35
ACSM. *See* American College of Sports Medicine
  activity questionnaire
  for diabetic athletes 246-250
  results 64-73
Actos 34
ADA. *See* American Diabetes Association
adenosine triphosphate (ATP) 16-22, 16*f*
adrenaline. *See* epinephrine
aerobic conditioning machines 166-171, 170*t*
aerobic dance 166-171, 170*t*
aerobic exercise components 4-10
  duration 8-9
  frequency 9-10
  intensity 6-8, 7*t*, 8*t*
  mode 5
  progression 10
aerobic energy system 20-22, 52, 89, 159, 160, 187. *See also* specific sports
aerobic workout components 12-13, 13*f*
aerobics. *See* aerobic dance
aerobics, water or aqua 166, 167*t*
aging 3, 5
altitude, exercise at 190, 195, 196, 239-242
Amaryl 34
American College of Sports Medicine (ACSM) 243
  exercise prescription 4-10
  type 1 diabetes and exercise 63-73, 64*t*
  type 2 diabetes and exercise 79-84
American Diabetes Association (ADA) 243
  type 1 diabetes and exercise 63-73, 64*t*, 75-78
  type 2 diabetes and exercise 79-84
amino acids 41-44, 43*t*

anaerobic energy systems 16-20
anaerobic glycolysis 17-18, 19*f*
antioxidant vitamins 47-49, 48*f*
aqua aerobics 166, 167*t*
arrhythmias 12, 78, 80, 84
athlete examples. *See* specific sports
athlete profiles
  Bill Talbert, tennis 56
  Bobby Clarke, ice hockey 85
  Chris Dudley, basketball 25
  Michelle McGann, golf 11
  Steve Prosterman, scuba 71
  Zippora Karz, ballet 39
ATP (adenosine triphosphate) 16-22, 16*f*
ATP-CP energy system 16-17, 17*f*, 52, 53, 134, 187. *See* specific sports
autonomic neuropathy 74, 76, 78, 80, 82, 84
Avandia 34

B

backpacking 190-196, 192*t*
badminton 223-225, 224*t*
ballet 236-237, 237*t*
ballroom dance 236-237, 237*t*
baseball 142-144, 143*t*
basketball 137-139, 138*t*
beach volleyball 218
benefits of exercise 3-4, 78, 81
beta-blockers and heart rate 6
bicycling. *See* cycling
blood sugars
  monitoring 66-67, 74, 82
  normal range 37
  variables affecting exercise 15
boating. *See* sailing
boogieboarding 208-210, 209*t*
bowling 238
boxing 182-183

about the author

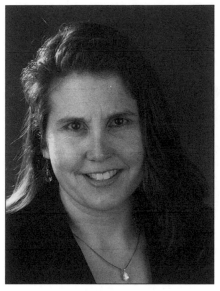

Sheri R. Colberg is an assistant professor of exercise science in the department of exercise science, physical education and recreation at Old Dominion University in Norfolk, Virginia. She holds a PhD in exercise physiology from the University of California at Berkeley, where she specialized in the areas of glucose and exercise metabolism and diabetes. She continues to conduct extensive research in these areas thanks to funding from sources including the American Diabetes Association.

Dr. Colberg has 32 years of practical experience as a type 1 diabetic athlete. As a certified exercise test technologist with the American College of Sports Medicine, she worked as an exercise specialist for a diabetes treatment center in San Francisco. She is a fellow of the American College of Sports Medicine, where she serves on the Professional Education and Ad Hoc Distance Learning Committees. She is also a professional member of the American Diabetes Association and former chair of the research section of the Virginia Association of Health, Physical Education, and Recreation.

Dr. Colberg lives in Virginia Beach with her husband and their three boys. She enjoys swimming, biking, walking, weight training, and yardwork, as well as playing with her three sons.